HOW TO HAVE A BABY AND STAY SANE

Virginia Ironside

Illustrated by
Christopher Ironside

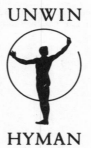

UNWIN

HYMAN

LONDON SYDNEY WELLINGTON

First published in Great Britain by the Trade Division of Unwin Hyman
Limited in 1989

UNWIN HYMAN LIMITED
15–17 Broadwick Street, London W1V 1FP

Allen & Unwin Australia Pty Ltd
8 Napier Street, North Sydney, NSW 2060, Australia

Allen & Unwin New Zealand Pty Ltd with the Port Nicholson Press
Compusales Building, 75 Ghuznee Street, Wellington, New Zealand

---

British Library Cataloguing in Publication Data

Ironside, Virginia
  How to have a baby and stay sane.
1. Babies. Home care
I. Title
649'.122

ISBN 0-04-440316-X

Typeset in 10 on 11 point Garamond by Nene Phototypesetters Ltd
and printed in Great Britain by Billing & Son, Worcester

Contents

Acknowledgements

With grateful thanks to Mirabel Cecil, Annette Stephens and, of course, Robin Grove-White.

Introduction

The first thing I remember about having a baby is the gooey sentimentality that surrounded the whole performance. I don't mean that my family was hovering over me with pale blue boottees; they weren't. But every book I read mentioned my 'little miracle' and emphasised the wonderful hours I would have playing with my baby, developing a warm and wonderful relationship with him and basking in the delight of my growing maternal instinct. Most books predicted an orgasmic birth that I would remember for the rest of my life, a fiercely protective and growing love for my small wonder and an ever-changing delight in watching him develop.

True, these feelings did pop up from time to time and very nice they were, too – but most often they didn't.

It was at four in the morning when my baby was eighteen months, still screaming three times a night, still breast-feeding, still howling when I left the room, still going to sleep at eleven p.m. and waking at five a.m., still not eating so much as a mashed banana . . . at a time when I was down to eight stone, had never had more than four hours sleep a night for a year and a half . . . it was then that I resolved that I'd put the record straight.

Because hunt as I might through the baby books – propping open my exhausted eyes with cotton buds – I found that the experts had only given half the picture about having babies. This is the other half.

And incidentally, if you're interested, yes, babies do stop waking and screaming and clinging and not eating. They develop all kinds of other peculiar and irritating habits, like everyone else, but on the whole babies, from the day they are born, just get better and better. Of course, you might argue, they couldn't get worse. My son is now the core of my eye and the apple of my life – and you can say what you like about my metaphors but don't dare criticise my child. But even all this love I feel for him now can't blot out the memory of those extraordinary days when he was tiny.

Here, then, is what I hope is an honest and lighthearted look at the strange, painful, joyful, miserable and happy experience of having a baby.

P.S. The reason I've called the baby 'he' throughout is because I had a boy and it came most naturally to me. And 'he' is quicker to type than 'she'.

1

Getting – and not Getting – Pregnant

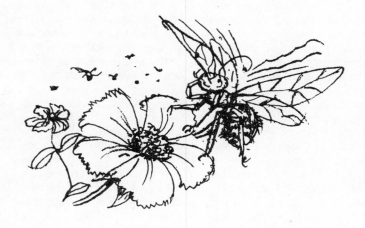

Whenever you make the mistake of telling anyone with children that you're thinking of starting a family the usual reaction is a spontaneous 'You must be mad!' This tactless phrase which has spontaneously slipped from their lips is usually followed up with smarmy apologies and lots of 'How wonderful for both of you' and 'Oh, at last you'll be a proper family' and 'Your parents will be so glad', and so on.

What they *mean* is: 'You must be mad.'

If you mention to your doctor the fact that you're thinking of trying for a baby, hoping to learn a bit about the sort of diet you ought to be eating, whether you should stop drinking and smoking before you even conceive, whether you can start trying to conceive the minute you come off the Pill, she will probably say, unnervingly: 'And *why* have you decided to have a baby?' She'll also ask how your partner feels about it, and all kinds of other personal questions that you don't want to answer.

The mature view is that you should only have a baby after much consideration, when both of you are certain that's what you want, when you've been in a relationship sufficiently long to know that it's likely to remain intact at least for the foreseeable year, and so on.

But people have babies for lots of very different reasons. Sometimes a woman is lonely or unemployed and feels useless at home all day when her partner is out at work – a perfectly valid reason for having a baby, I'd say, but not everyone agrees. Some partnerships are fairly rocky and feel a baby might help glue it together. This is risky as an idea, but there's no question it does work in many cases. Marriage guidance counsellors and agony aunts, after all, so often recommend finding 'shared interests' to heal an ailing marriage; and what is a child but a shared interest? You couldn't find anything more shared; you couldn't find anything more interesting. Not only that, but having children does make it a lot more difficult to split up. Most people do have children to bind them together for ever – and even if they divorce, this is usually the case. Marriage is easily dissolved by divorce; shared parenthood can never, ever be broken. Some people want to have a baby just to see if they're fertile or not.

Most people decide to have a baby simply because they love the idea of looking after a little person – the urge to nurture is strong in both men and women as they mature – and others have children because each partner longs either to put right an unhappy childhood second-hand, so to speak, or to relive, vicariously, their own happy childhoods. I was always surprised to find how much I enjoyed sharing childhood activities with my son – from swimming, to going to museums, to eating ice-creams, going to the circus and even reading *Winnie the Pooh*. Many parents enjoy every minute of childish fun, almost as much as and sometimes more than their children, a fact that they often seek to conceal out of a misguided sense of shame that they find childish things such good fun. I would love to have made clothes for a daughter's doll; I enjoyed, instead, colouring, magic-painting, invisible pictures and making Lego models; my son's father liked romping around with him, taking him to the zoo and so on – all activities that neither of us would have been likely to have done either on our own or as a childless couple.

Some couples – men, perhaps, more than women – want to have children to continue some family line; they want to leave something of their own behind them to carry on the good work, be it banking or burgling. Other couples aren't sure what they want so they leave the whole thing to chance to avoid having to take a decision about it. As playing Russian roulette with contraceptives invariably leads to pregnancy in the end, fate doesn't play much of a part. But if it makes everyone feel happier that fate has decided the pregnancy rather than they themselves (which is what really has happened), then fair enough. Sometimes it's a good idea to kid yourself.

Some women try to get pregnant beause they fear that if they leave it any later they might be over the hill. And since the risk of having handicapped children is far greater over the age of thirty-five and the chances of getting pregnant reduce dramatically after the age of thirty-five – over a third of women at forty are infertile just because of their age – that's another good reason to go ahead.

How on earth can you weigh up the pros and cons of having a child, for heaven's sake, if you've never had one before? All decisions to have a first child are wild leaps in the dark. No amount of thought or counselling will help you come to a mature decision.

Most women do tend to expect they'll get pregnant the first month they throw away their diapraghm or stop taking the Pill. But in fact you don't get infertility investigations until you've been trying for a year – unless you are over thirty-five, in which case it is six months – which is the time by which the vast majority of couples will have conceived.

However, you can speed up your chances of getting pregnant, and if you're one of those women who once they decide to get pregnant find themselves in floods of tears the moment a period comes on, then it's well worth taking the trouble. The time you're most fertile is fourteen days before your period. As sperm can live in your body for a few days you should start to have sex a day or so before you ovulate. You can find out when you ovulate by asking your local Family Planning Association for a temperature chart which gives you all the information; or there are also more sophisticated ovulation prediction kits you can buy at chemists. Timing is a cold-blooded but efficient method and does involve your partner's co-operation. If he starts complaining of feeling like a stud, do remind him that you feel just the same only like a breeding machine. And if you can screw yourself up to having sex on certain days, whether you feel like it or not, he ought at least to have the decency to have a good try as well. If he tries and fails, then that's another matter.

However, you may be fairly certain that you can get pregnant quickly. You may be so confident, in fact, that you'd like to try to get a baby of the sex you prefer. Most parents don't mind that much about the sex of the first baby and if you have a sneaking feeling that your husband would prefer a boy, don't count on it: lots of fathers are scared stiff of having boys. Indeed, some men feel extremely threatened by the idea of having another man around the house, albeit that that man is only eighteen inches long, bald, red-faced and wears nappies.

But if you're agreed on trying for a certain sex, you can go ahead. The theory goes that the maleness or femaleness of a baby is determined by the sperm, not the egg. According to one school of thought, a tendency to acidity in the balance of the blood in males produces more female sperm. So if you want a girl, your man must jog and lift weights until he's blue in the face. A more sedentary life results in more male sperm being around, so sit him down if you want a boy. Male sperm are more vigorous than female ones (and they die quicker – just as men do in adult life!), therefore if you want a boy, time intercourse to the day of ovulation when the male sperm will hare up the tubes and get there first. For a girl, time your intercourse a couple of days before you ovulate. By the time the egg arrives the male sperm will be dead and the females can wend their ladylike way up to the egg.

Similarly, a woman who douches with a mixture of two tablespoons of

3

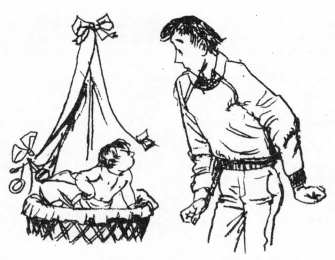

'Indeed, some men feel extremely threatened by the idea of having another man about the house'

white vinegar to a quart of water will encourage female sperm. To encourage male ones, douche with two tablespoons of baking soda to a quart of water. All this is highly unorthodox, I might add, and totally unproven by scientific research.

Once you miss a period you may well be pregnant. In fact, if you feel a bit unlike your usual self before you've missed a period, with especially tender breasts and a bloated feeling in your body, you might like to try one of the home pregnancy testing kits that can give incredibly early results. All this involves tinkering around with a wonderfully delicate little kit which should give you a quick result. You sit on the loo feeling like a mad scientist as you drip your morning urine into a test tube (more of the pregnancy hormone has accumulated over the night than during the day), shake it around, and leave it on its little mirrored stand until the time is up. The advantage of a home pregnancy test is that you can do it earlier than a test at the doctor, and you don't feel such a twit as you hear endless negative results via your doctor's receptionist.

Eventually, I hope, you get your good news. Or is it good news? To travel hopefully is sometimes better than to arrive and when that test shows you are indeed pregnant, your reactions can be unpredictable. Some mothers experience a surge of emotion flooding over them as they realise they're fertile, bearing the child of the man they love, with their genes living on for generation after generation, at last fitting into the world's great life-cycle. Others may be unable to take in the good news; others (no less admirable than the former) may well be appalled to find that not a single massed choir or violin do they hear, heralding the good news into their innermost soul – only a faint whiff of sheer panic.

4

It's no use bleating: 'But I didn't *mean* it! I want to think about it rather more carefully! Put the clock back!' As my rotund ante-natal teacher used to say, with a rather wolf-like smile: 'It's too late now to do anything. You're having a baby. It's not like a new pair of shoes. If you don't like it, you can't take it back to the shops!'

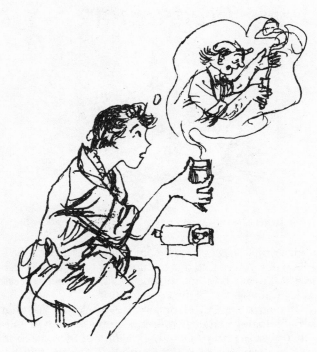

'You sit on the loo feeling like a mad scientist'

2

Pregnancy

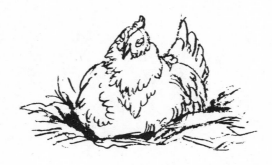

The first hint you'll have of the completely disorientating state of pregnancy is when you're told that the duration of pregnancy is not nine months, as we were all told at school, but in fact forty weeks or, rather, ten lunar months from the date of the last period.

From then on in, be prepared for surprises every day. Your figure will slowly alter completely; other people's perceptions of you will change dramatically (on being pregnant you'll become secondary to this new, important, invader inside you), your moods and tastes will be turned upside down by excesses of hormones and you'll be plunged for the next few years of your life into a strange new world, clutching your baby books in a vain attempt to find some reason in all the madness.

One of the most disorientating aspects of pregnancy for most of us who, particularly these days, have very little experience of pregnancy or babies in our adult lives, is the sense of the unknown. In some ways it's like entering a ghost train at a funfair. However much you tell yourself that everyone who has been on it before has come out unscathed, however much you reason that it's unlikely that the owners of the fairground would have picked you to test a new route that might drive you mad or kill you half way through, the first time is always frightening. Will you have changed when you emerge the other side? Do you *want* to change? Could you cope? And nothing adds more to the confusion than your own body in the early stages; because although you yourself may be bursting with joy in the early months, physically you'll be flat as a board.

There's no tangible evidence of this mysterious baby. You can, bafflingly, get into all your usual clothes. You've only got your doctor's word for it that you're pregnant at all – and the fact that most likely you'll feel permanently queasy.

In many ways it's an enormous relief when the day comes, around the fourth month, that your stomach actually begins to assume if not football, at least tennis ball proportions . . . and at last you can justifiably clamber into those floppy smocks, stick your feet into sensible sandals and Be Pregnant.

Now, despite much reassurance that pregnancy is 'natural' and therefore shouldn't hurt or be uncomfortable (notice that no one ever makes such claims for dying, equally natural), it's common to suffer a fair amount during pregnancy. From day one you must remember that for most women, pregnancy has it's unpleasant aspects. Between the idea that 'Everything's fine' and, on the other hand, 'Everything's ghastly' is some kind of truth. On the bad side, insomnia, backache, piles, heartburn, exhaustion, constipation, morning sickness, bleeding gums, thrush, varicose veins, cramps and palpitations are among the many expected symptoms of pregnancy. More serious are toxaemia (a form of blood-poisoning), anaemia and possible miscarriage. Indeed, it's only in this last century that a possibility of death itself for you, the mother, has been struck off the list of realistic dangers.

Feeling grim some of the time is a 'natural' part of 'natural' pregnancy. But so, too, is feeling wonderful. And you should be able to look forward, also, to periods when you do feel serene, when your skin glows and your hair shines and you smile like a Buddha.

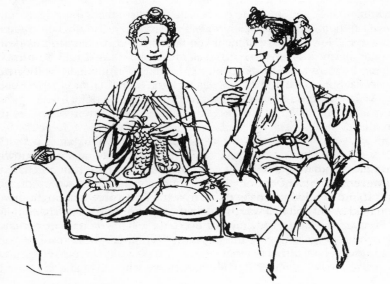

Because of your altered hormonal structure you'll *feel* different as a personality as well. For the first few months you may find your emotions have more in common with an Italian opera singer than an English rose. (From not giving a pin about Britain or how great she was, I found myself bursting into tears every time I heard the National Anthem.)

So avoid all possible areas of conflict. Don't wait until screaming point as your father-in-law tells you, yet again, about the great match between Arsenal and Chelsea in 1949 – go to bed. Don't risk not getting your job back later by threatening suicide every time you're asked to make more than a simple phone call – get as good a deal as you can out of your employer and leave. Better to demand to sit down on those 'seats designed for handicapped people' in the bus, than collapse on the way home.

Be prepared, too, for craving some special and unlikely dish; winter strawberries or asparagus, for example (nearly all mums seem to crave something rare and expensive, thus making their 'craving' credibility low in the eyes of men. But would he rather sit and watch you chewing coal over the supper table – as some mums have done?) You may also become sickened by familiar tastes and smells. Even some special soap that you've been buying for years as a treat may suddenly make you want to throw up as if it were an old putrifying fish sitting on your basin. Get rid of it. If you have to, move out of your temporarily stinking house for a few days.

As far as diet goes there's a lot of conflicting information. Should you take extra vitamins? No, not unless your doctor advises you to because of your disgustingly unhealthy diet of crisps, chips, chip butties followed by toast, swilled down with gallons of Coca-Cola day after day after day. Better, anyway, to switch to a more sensible diet than to take extra vitamins which can, in some cases, actually harm the baby if you go to town on them. Obviously pills and drugs should generally be avoided, but there's no evidence that the odd mild painkiller like paracetamol will do any harm at all in early pregnancy. Should you drink? The latest research seems to show that around 1½ units of drink a day will do no harm – a unit is a small sherry, a glass of wine or half a pint of beer. But if you've been out on a binge you shouldn't worry. Just don't make a habit of it and, best of all, avoid excess alcohol consumption when you're pregnant.

Every woman must know that it's wisest to give up smoking – but there are some organisations that give really alarmist advice on what's known as preconceptual care, insisting, even, that you must be serene and happy all through pregnancy because, they claim, any shock or sad event can have a profound effect on the unborn foetus. In my view this is complete poppycock and there has been no conclusive research on this *at all*.

Pregnancy is never the same for two people. One woman may spend the whole pregnancy sick and depressed; another will be radiant and euphoric with maternal feelings. Some women really do feel serene and look like ads for skin tonic while they move with curious grace under

Laura Ashley smocks; others feel ill and miserable from Day One, their skin goes blotchy, their legs swell up, they're sick every morning and look like sacks of potatoes on sticks. What is 'radiant' for one is 'cow-like' for another.

Serene or slutty, there's no mother who doesn't feel extremely uncomfortable during the last few months – and you will too. The extra weight of the baby is heavy and cumbersome and even your bone structure is having to shift slightly to accommodate the child, often producing odd aches here and there. There's little point, at this stage, in doing anything except making life more comfortable for yourself. If you feel too awful, simply go to bed at nine every night. The Pregnant Walk must be overcome. Flat, unattractive (but incredibly comfortable) shoes

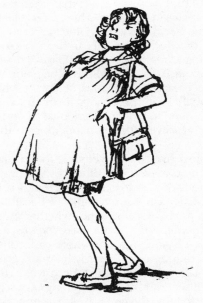

'The Pregnant Walk'

must be bought. You must remove your hand from its permanent position in the small of your aching back and straighten your spine, now curved like a bow as you stare at the sky, trying to balance the huge lump suspended in front. You must learn, too, to grab for comfort, particularly in all your friends' sitting-rooms which suddenly reveal themselves as being excruciatingly uncomfortable – except, of course, the one chair in which the friend himself always sits. An evening at the theatre will be marred by sitting scrunched up in a tiny seat for three hours. One way to get relief is to wallow in a bath with the water supporting the baby. If you go on holiday, go to the seaside and borrow a pregnancy bathing-suit. At home, oil your skin (never proved as at all useful in lessening stretch marks, but just a luxury in itself), before taking up your patchwork to stitch a lining for your Moses basket. It may sound soppy but it's a better way of spending an evening than out with friends at a minute bistro, rammed into a tiny seat, choking on cigarette smoke and unable to keep your eyes open with fatigue.

The fatigue comes not only because of the exhaustion of carrying that weight around everywhere, but also because it's often hard to sleep at night. Sometimes you can't sleep for worry. As your womb enlarges so do your fantasies about what's inside. Because the baby is growing inside *you*, outsiders tend to feel that you've got some special knowledge of your unborn child. You are a Mother and you contain Mother's Secret inside you. It's as if they almost suspect that when they aren't there, you let the baby out for runs in private and have a few laughs with it. But *your* fear comes from the fact that Mother's Little Secret is also secret from *you*. Despite feelings of affection to this unborn person, you'll also feel moments of alarm and fear about this unknown creature that is feeding within you. And because of your feelings of affection you'd also be pretty inhuman not to feel extremely anxious, at least at some moments, about whether it's 'normal'. From pregnancy through to babyhood it's fairly common for mothers to suffer occasional X-certificate nightmares involving, usually, terrifying things happening to their child, born or unborn.

If you're over thirty-five you'll be eligible for an amniocentesis, which should put your mind at rest. The fluid that surrounds the baby in the womb is the amniotic fluid and contains the baby's urine and living cells shed from the baby's skin. So a sample of this fluid can give lots of information about the baby, for instance whether it suffers from Down's Syndrome. If you have this test, don't make the mistake of going without taking along a friend. Although the whole procedure doesn't actually hurt, women generally agree it's a fairly hairy experience. As one mum put it, it's not so much the night of the long knives as the afternoon of the long needle. You'll see everything happening on a screen, including the needle being inserted into the amniotic sac to draw off some of the fluid to be tested, and after some weeks you'll know whether the baby is okay or not.

This test does reveal the sex of the baby so if you want to be in on what should surely be your secret just as much as the doctor's, then make sure the hospital is prepared to give you the information before you go ahead with the test. Some hospitals, unbelievably, actually refuse to divulge this information, even if you beg them.

Assuming the amniocentesis has set your mind at rest, insomnia can still arise for a purely practical reason – the baby's squirming, hiccuping and kicking. It seems as if it's been rocked to sleep by lolling around the water of the womb as you tottered about during the day, then springs into

10

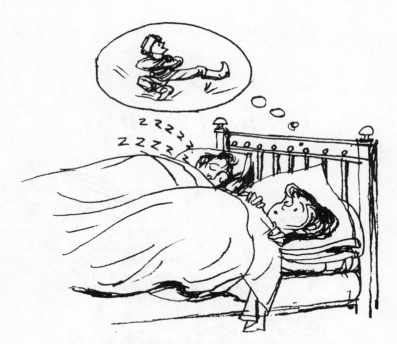

'Performing a Cossack dance from your ribs down to your hip bones'

action at night, kicking up half-formed heels, putting on tiny dancin' shoes and performing a Cossack dance from your ribs down to your hip bones. In fact babies move all the time; it's just that you notice the movement more at night. It's worth defying grumbles from your partner and surrounding yourself with pillows. (Caruso slept every night with eighteen pillows and he wasn't pregnant, just fat.) And remember not to drink too much liquid before going to bed. From the beginning of pregnancy you'll need to pee more than usual and at the end of the pregnancy the baby's head presses on the bladder, adding to the problem so that you can hardly hold more than a tablespoon of pee before you have to run for the loo.

If you're obeying your doctor's orders as you should be and, on top of all this suffering, are not drinking too much, not smoking and not taking any pills that haven't been approved by him, you'll probably be counting off the days to when you can give birth and get back to normal life. You can make these days go quicker by getting prepared, both psychologically and practically, for the birth itself.

3

Getting Prepared

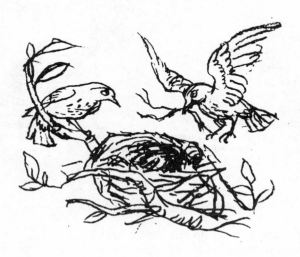

Although its always hard to get pregnancy into proportion – it's common to pretend either that the baby just isn't there or to become an obsessive baby-addict from Day One – being prepared is what pregnancy is all about. And although it's important to have something else to think about during pregnancy other than babies, it's well worth taking the time to save yourself unnecessary misery and agony later on. As a first-time mum you really would be sensible to have your baby in hospital, Just in Case. But as the hospital takes precautionary measures against possible disaster, follow its example and take precautionary measures against a possible bad hospital.

But which hospital? The questions to ask are:

1   Is it policy to allow husbands, partners or friends in to attend and help with the birth? 'Hubbies' (for so they are called by the hospital staff until delivery when they become 'dads'; you are, however, 'mother' and the baby is 'baby' from the beginning of labour) – 'hubbies' do come into their own during labour. Since there are still

hospitals which discourage the presence of partners (to the extent that only rudeness and force will persuade them to let them in), it's important to find out what the policy is before you get to the hospital.

2   Are epidurals available? These are injections of local anaesthetic into the space between the spine and the backbone.

3   Are inductions given against your wishes? An induction means that the birth of the baby is induced early by means of drugs, a process which can be essential in some cases. (No hospital would admit to this, but it's always best to make your position clear before you go in. Your position, unless you particularly want your baby to be born at a certain time, is that you do *not* want an induction unless you can be convinced that it's a medical necessity.)

4   Is the policy to shave off all your pubic hair before birth? (Completely unnecessary according to some reports and most tickly, scratchy, embarrassing and uncomfortable according to *all* reports.)

5   Is an enema or a suppository given on your entrance to the hospital? (Both are extremely unpleasant, but a suppository is the least unpleasant since it is a long pill-like object you can insert yourself, while an enema is a fluid that has to be injected up you by a nurse.)

6   Is the hospital reasonably open-minded about the way you give birth? Some mums like to be able to move around during birth and give birth standing or bending. Some hospitals regard this as out of the question.

7   Are episiotomies automatically performed? An episiotomy is a small cut made at the entrance of your vagina to stop it tearing when the baby emerges. Of course it doesn't always tear, but some doctors feel it's best to be on the safe side because cuts are easier to repair than tears. (There are good arguments both for and against them, so read up about it, ask around and find out where your hospital stands on the issue.)

8   If they do episiotomies, are they stitched with soluble thread? (If so, the stitches will drop out into your bed and the doctors won't have to remove them after the birth, a particularly ouch-making procedure.)

9   Are the visiting hours lax? (Some mums love this; others prefer to be sheltered from the entire typing-pool arriving in the middle of their afternoon naps with plastic ducks, grapes and boottees.)

10   Is the baby allowed to be by your side all the time (if you wish) and at the same time will the staff take it away to feed it in the nursery for nights or days (if you wish)?

11   Is breast-feeding looked down on as a thorough nuisance only taken up by long-skirted, barefoot poetesses from Hampstead, or is it up to you whether you breast- or bottle-feed?

12   If you wish to breast-feed can you be sure of help and encouragement?

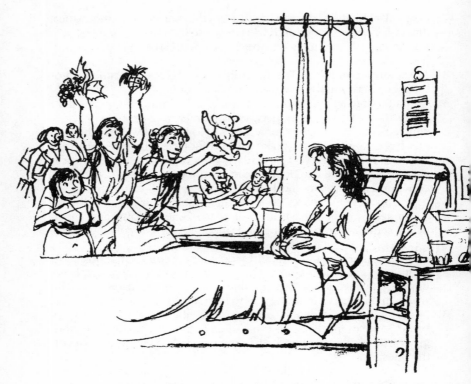

'Others prefer to be sheltered from the entire typing-pool'

A foretaste of what's to come can be gleaned from your innumerable visits to the ante-natal clinic. If it's more anti than ante, then change. There's no point in putting up with long waits sitting on uncomfortable institutional chairs, reading old copies of *Mother and Baby*, surrounded by a collection of drawn, worn and tired mums with bulging stomachs, often with two or three kids already in tow.

Why suffer hardly ever seeing the same doctor twice and running the whole gamut from the friendly woman who warms her stethoscope before applying it to the football in your abdomen and allows you to listen to your baby's heart-beat (you never can hear it; just be polite and pretend) – to the grim-faced consultant who looks at you (and every other pregnant woman) with that particular glance of disgust, pity and dismissal that is all too common in senior obstetricians?

Ante-natal clinics have improved vastly recently and if you ask intelligent questions you should expect to get intelligent answers. It's foolish to go home in tears because the obstetrician frowned when he felt your bump when you could have saved days of misery by asking, 'Why are you frowning?' He may well have frowned because he had a row with his wife that morning, not because he suspects that you are bearing a two-headed hydra (in which case, being an obstetrician, his face would more likely be aglow with lively interest).

Incidentally, a combination of internal examinations by white-coated strangers, unbalanced hormones and sheer fatigue can have a disastrous effect on your sex-life since every time you strip off and lie panting on your bed, you are instantly reminded of the clinic. If your doctor has any reservations about sex at certain times in your case, fine; but actually there's nothing to prove that sex is harmful in general. Your size is the only turn-off, but some couples keep going with sex until the last day by means of compasses, graphs and Ordnance Survey maps. It must be said, however, that lots of women don't feel like it on the grounds that it seems, suddenly, pointless.

The clinic not only checks that the baby is growing at the proper rate; it also keeps you, quite rightly, in a permanent state of alarm about blood pressure. This is important because if it does go up you might well be doomed to spend weeks in the mother-to-be's prison, the ante-natal ward, where fat women with red cheeks and racing hearts slag around in slippers and dressing-gowns all day 'resting' to get the pressure down so that they can be allowed home.

In between your ante-natal visits you must flap along to the shops in your flat shoes to assemble the layette and buy a feeding bra. While

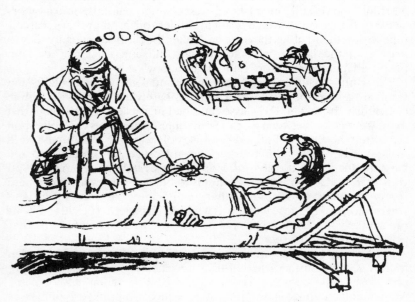

'He may well have frowned because he had a row with his wife that morning'

indeed it may be true, as experienced mums will tell you, that the baby can sleep in the bottom drawer of the chest of drawers, the washing-up basin can double up as a bath, the Babygros can be bought at jumble sales and your cousin could provide you with her old carrycot, there's no question that you as a new mother will wish to Do Everything Right. That casual approach and welcoming of hand-me-downs will be reserved for the second and third child. Now you are confronted in the shops by a baffling display of baby-jumpers, cots, wheels, springing chairs, harnesses and nappy-changers. Rightly, you suspect that you are being conned. At one of the most vulnerable stages in your life, when women in your condition are rarely found guilty of shop-lifting (which shows what the law thinks of your mental state), you are presented with a glittering array of so-called 'necessities' which appeal to your maternal instinct or your guilt (for your lack of maternal instinct). I would make a list of what you feel are the barest essentials and then cut them down to half. You can always buy them later.

The next step is to prepare yourself for the birth. Although until recently it was fashionable to believe that virtually painless childbirth could be achieved if the mother were sufficiently 'relaxed', the method of relaxing, known as psychoprophylaxis, has lost some credibility these days – not least as a result of mothers who tried the relaxing method, practised their exercises every day, learnt a little jingle off by heart to repeat to themselves during contractions and who forced their partners to simulate labour pains at home by getting them to pinch their legs black and blue, and yet still found labour excruciatingly painful. Some mothers swear by the exercises which result in painless birth; others have scarcely time to give their babies the once-over after the birth so eager are they to leap from the labour table to strangle the ante-natal teacher who promised mere 'discomfort' rather than 'agony'.

The truth is that some births are agony and some are marvellous and some are a bit of both, and 'relaxing' has barely anything to do with it. (Obviously those who did classes and had marvellous births claim that there *is* a relation between them.) Some ante-natal classes can quite spoil the birth with their unfulfilled promises of ease and 'naturalness', and make mothers who don't experience pleasure feel guilty into the bargain. But classes do offer other advantages. Attending them gives you your first chance to meet other mums-to-be and, however reticent and reserved you are, a gossip with others in the same boat is reassuring. And you're accepted by these women as well, which is a relief because in your private life you may well have been dismayed by the alteration in other people's attitudes to you.

'Nudge, nudge, wink, wink' remarks made to your partner by his men friends, or the immediate intimacy revealed by women who were previously quite cool and reserved, can be very irritating. For some women think nothing of dropping all reticence, whipping up your jersey to stare at your tummy and making leering remarks like, 'Oooh, you don't

16

know what you're in for! No more career for you! You're going to turn into a vegetable like the rest of us! No more going to the movies, no more sex in the afternoons, ha ha!' 'Make the most of your life now because you won't have any time for yourself for the rest of it! Now you're done for!' 'And aren't you absolutely terrified of the birth? Well my dear, you should be. My labour went on for three days and three nights, and the doctor said . . .'

Apart from providing new and more sympathetic friends, classes are a good way of acquiring information about birth as well. And clearly an informed and confident approach to birth, while by no means preventing pain, has some beneficial effects, if only for morale boosting.

Ante-natal classes nearly always arrange 'dad's night' too, near the end of the pregnancy. All 'dads', even the dad you love, appear scarlet with embarrassment, looking like characters out of American domestic comedies, twisting their hands, tripping over their feet and asking barmy questions about the technical side of birth. They all look extremely small and weedy compared with the pregnant giantesses that are their wives. However a 'dad' who knows how to massage your back for twelve hours on end, hold your hand, press the emergency button and mop your brow with a cool sponge, really is a help as far as the pain and discomfort go.

Some weeks before your expected delivery date you will probably have already started packing a little suitcase to take with you into hospital. You may think you're crazy to be so well-prepared, but this is what the nesting instinct does for you. On top of all the personal things you know you'll need, I suggest you add the following:

- Flannel and sponge (for your partner to mop your brow with during labour).
- Instamatic camera (for your partner to take pictures with during the birth).
- Food and drink (so your partner can have a snack on the spot if he gets hungry).
- One very old nightdress (to wear immediately after you've given birth. If you wear your prettiest nightie the minute you get into the ward after giving birth you may well find it covered with blood the following morning).
- Slippers, toothbrush, toothpaste, two nightdresses that open in the front (if you want to breast-feed).
- Two to three nursing bras.
- Glucose tablets for energy.
- Supply of ten-pence bits for anxious phone calls.
- Stamps, envelopes, writing paper (to thank all those relations for sending those inevitable yellow Acrilan play-suits for the baby).
- Cologne spray to cool you down during labour and in hospital afterwards.
- Detergent (to do your washing with).

- *Do-it-Yourself Relief Kit*, consisting of tissues; Vaseline for sore bits; over-the-counter painkillers of your own (so you're not constantly badgering sulky night-nurses at four in the morning); anaesthetic spray (essential for giving local relief, particularly with pain from an episiotomy scar); Senakot tablets (try dosing yourself with these if you get constipated after birth – which you almost certainly will – before you resort to begging for suppositories or enemas. Doesn't affect the baby via your milk, incidentally.)

Armed with this kit you won't have to suffer any nights waiting in agony before you can assign your friends to drop medicaments in the following day.

Although most women suffer a kind of stage-fright about three to six weeks before the birth, luckily for them Nature usually contrives to make first babies late. Enough friends ringing up in the middle of your afternoon nap to ask: 'Are you *still* at home?' (it's worth taking the phone off the hook during the last days, incidentally) and the extra discomfort of the last few days are enough to make most women positively long for birth. Pregnancy has finally become intolerable. And so it is that you, like most women, will enter hospital not in fear, but in relief. Hospital no longer seems frightening. 'Come unto me all ye who labour and are heavy laden,' it seems to say, 'and I will give you rest.'

4

Birth

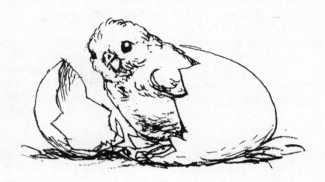

The most important aspect of birth is the entrance into your life of a new lodger with a ninety-nine year lease in his hands – and the realisation that from now on you've turned into one of life's landladies: cooking breakfast, making beds and fixing bath routines for the next ten years at least. Yet this aspect, about which there should be many genuine worries, is always overshadowed by the actual birth itself. The painful side of birth, in particular, has always been given particular priority.

Considering a birth takes about a day and that you'll be slaving for, or certainly thinking about, your child at some point every day for the next twenty years at least, an awful lot of fuss is made about the actual birth – particularly as it has been endured by millions and millions of times over millions and millions of years by millions and millions of women far more cowardly and stupid than you. Indeed 242 women give birth every minute throughout the world. For hundreds of years women have been terrified by old wives' tales of blood, gore, rips, tears, screams, sweat and agony. In the last decade women have been fed a completely *new* wives' tale: that birth should be bliss, that it should be a wonderful, sensual, indeed almost orgasmic experience and that the only pain connected with it is the mother's own fault (for being hung-up, neurotic or uneducated). This is just as much of a fiction as the first – and brings with it a lot of shame, misery and guilt, too.

Primitive women, argue the 'birth is bliss' brigade, feel no pain; they just go off into a field and have their babies. But you might remember that no one has yet questioned the primitive woman. It has been suggested that primitive women go off into the field and scream their heads off. It's also reported that many women of different cultures have *apparently* painless births because of strict social taboos (for instance, if they scream it's a sure sign they've been unfaithful to their husbands, which is enough to silence most mums at this crucial stage. They've got enough to worry about without divorce.)

There is actually no evidence that primitive women have any better a time than we do. Of course all the complications involved these days in saving babies who would otherwise have died or suffered brain damage – forceps, caesarians, etc. – mean that we have to pay a price in pain for saving them (and, often, our own lives). The commonly used induction (which involves an artificial rupture of the membranes and a pessary which stimulates the uterus to contract more strongly), is claimed by some women to result in a slightly more painful birth than a natural one – but saves the lives of hundreds of babies which might otherwise die in the uterus.

Rather than anticipate only pain or bliss, it's much better to approach birth realistically. It might be painless; it might be bliss; it might be neither. Whatever it is, luckily for us, living in these liberated and medically advanced times, *there's no need to suffer at all, if the doctor handles things correctly.*

Although relaxation classes have never been proved to reduce pain, their teaching to concentrate on a song or a spot on the wall can do much to inhibit pain (on the lines of 'Think hard of something else and then you won't notice it'). A general improvement in birth education and a social atmosphere that makes it easier to talk about birth in advance must take some credit for releasing the sort of pain induced by fear. Gas and air, given by all hospitals, is a blessing to all mothers, and epidurals, if available and properly administered, give complete relief. The disadvantage of epidurals, which knock you out from the waist down only, is that, although you are completely conscious and can watch everything happily, you can't feel yourself giving birth; but ideally you miss out all the pain as well.

The nicest way to give birth is, obviously, to *try* to have the baby 'naturally' because lots of mothers don't suffer unbearable pain. (I didn't, and put it all down to my relaxation classes until I heard what other mothers in my own class had to say!) *But* always have drugs and, at the last resort, an epidural on hand in case the whole thing does become agonising. Properly planned in advance there should, ideally, be no problem. Never feel that you're letting yourself down if you get desperate for pain relief; and remember that those who make the most fuss get most attention.

If the idea of modern drugs isn't enough of a reassurance do try to remember there have been rare cases of fifty-year-old grannies who, thinking their periods stopping is simply the change of life, suddenly come over all funny one day, lie down and find they've got a new baby in a couple of minutes. One eleven-year-old, so ashamed of her unmarried condition, was known to give birth alone at the top of a high-rise block of flats and was seen, perfectly healthy, wheeling a pram around a few days later. Although, in rare cases, labour can last twenty-four hours with a first baby, birth is by no means always an excruciatingly painful event.

There are three ways which signify you're about to give birth: you can have a show, your waters can break or you can get contractions. The very words of this pre-birth jargon can be alarming and you'll be no exception when you suspect that it won't be as simple as it says in the books. You fear that you'll be the only one who won't spot the symptoms, or that you'll start giving birth miles away from a hospital. (Many women, afraid that they'll be caught unawares, refuse all engagements for days before the expected date of delivery, dooming themselves to tedious nights of waiting which sometimes continue for a fortnight, reminiscent of nights as a teenager when they waited in misery evening after evening for Mr Right to ring. It's actually much better to book yourself well up even during the week you think you'll deliver. Like taking an umbrella out to prevent rain, being over-anxious about staying in always seems to prevent birth – it doesn't really, but it does seem like it.)

A 'show' is a spot of blood, like the beginning of a period; the 'waters' breaking (which always reminded me of the Red Sea parting) is simply a gush of fluid from the womb; and contractions, which feel something like the pains during the worst moments of gastric flu, are a sign that your muscles are getting into action for widening the exit for the baby to get out into the birth canal. You are in labour when these contractions are around fifteen minutes apart.

As a first-time mum you'll have lots of false alarms – but don't worry. It is impossible to mistake going into labour for anything else.

It's best to rely on an ambulance to take you to hospital if your partner plans to stay with you during the birth, because if he drives you he will emerge elated, about sixteen hours later, only to find his joy blighted by parking tickets and wheel-clamps.

Once at the hospital, you'll probably be put through a routine of the usual tests and be given a bath and a suppository (if it's a civilised place; otherwise an enema, arguably more unpleasant than the birth itself to prevent embarrassing scenes on the labour table and to make more room for the baby's exit). You'll also be examined to see how dilated your cervix is.

However prepared you are for pain, blood and thunder, you'll never be well-enough prepared for the loneliness and length of birth. Every film of a birth shows a highly edited version of the delivery (the producer has naturally cut out the boring bits). But for the first few hours that you're in the labour ward, suitably dressed in a regimental nightie, you'll most likely be alone, apart from the odd nurse popping in to check that you're not dying. Your body has, by this time, started to take over; contractions attack you and release you with a power you would never have dreamt you were capable of. Muscles you never knew you had start heaving into action. Uninhibited grunts and groans escape your lips.

This is the First Stage, as the cervix opens to release the baby into the birth canal. It's during these long hours that the ante-natal teacher will expect you and your husband to get out your crossword puzzles, discuss the domestic accounts or brush up on your backgammon, chatting blithely in between contractions. Old-timers who have had more than one baby (for as soon as you've had one baby you're an old-timer) may well be able to think of things other than birth during this time, but it's unlikely that any first mother would take kindly to a bit of knitting stuck into her hands at this stage.

At the beginning of the Second Stage, the pushing stage, the labour staff won't be satisfied with just popping in to check from time to time. They'll be on the alert. If you're in a teaching hospital, a fresh-faced young man looking barely old enough to be a policeman will come in and say, 'Hi, I'm Gerry/Al/Rodney and I'm going to deliver your baby,' which is a bit of a let-down when you've been imagining all along some wise old grey-haired doctor like Grantly Dick Read sitting by your bedside hour after hour.

This second stage is much quicker than the first stage, but much more alarming. The contractions become more powerful. The doctor might perform an episiotomy by cutting you slightly to prevent tearing. By now the midwives are starting to hover round and the whole room seems to be full of people with J-cloths on their heads. You may even have a male midwife if you're lucky. If none of them seem to be paying much attention, just standing around gossiping about shopping and the weather, welcome this as a sign of their professionalism – they've seen it all before, luckily for you. At this point in the delivery most mothers *do* wonder if they can stand it a minute longer. But just at the moment that it feels unendurable, the baby is born ... usually painlessly. The actual moment of delivery is never as painful as the build-up to it. Indeed, the actual moment of the birth is usually so painless that most mothers can only tell what's happening by the way their stomachs suddenly start to flatten into a heap of shuddering flesh looking wrinkly and wobbly, like a collapsed parachute. You will only know that you have given birth by the general cry of glee, 'hubby' (or, rather, 'dad' as he has now become) bursting into tears (and perhaps you, too): then you catch sight of something blue and slithery and miniscule being held up triumphantly by the midwife.

Men really do come into their own during the birth. If they're not so excited by the pregnancy, the birth is quite a different matter. Phrases like 'Marvellous!' and 'The most exciting moment of my life!', 'Mind-blowing!' abound. In all cultures men are pleasantly freaked-out by it all. There is

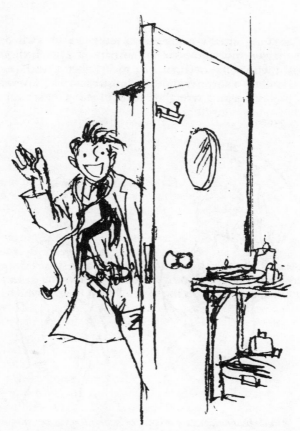

'Hi, I'm Gerry/Al/Rodney and I'm going to deliver your baby'

some primitive tribe where all the men go off in to the woods and have labour pains while their wives are giving birth – and there's something of that tribe in most British males, even the ones, I suspect, who have to get blind drunk with their mates while the birth is happening. They're not just carrying on as if nothing is happening, after all. Their friends are standing round them with support (in more ways than one, by closing time) in the same way as the women-folk are around the mother having the child.

You are likely to be a bit shocked by the appearance of your baby. A new baby is often blue, his head is a weird, long shape, like Nephertite's, narrowed to make it easier to get out, he has bow legs, his eyes are shut, he's covered in a white sticky stuff called vernix, usually mixed with blood and mucus, his genitalia may be swollen or an odd colour, he may have swollen breasts and be covered with unsightly body hair. It's best to get your husband to deny quickly that he looks like *his* side of the family at this stage, to stop any wrangling later. Whatever you feel – love, loathing or indifference (and all are equally natural feelings) – this will not be the baby you expected; not, necessarily, the baby you even thought you wanted. A baby who will grow up to be a male ballet-dancer, perhaps, or a small stockbroker, a stripper or a headmistress – who knows. But for now, just a tiny, squeaking wriggling handful still almost as much of a mystery as when it was inside you.

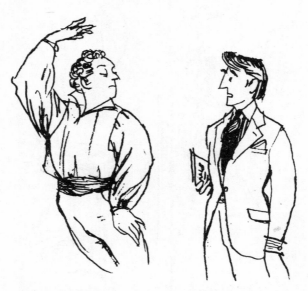

'A male ballet-dancer, perhaps, or a small stockbroker'

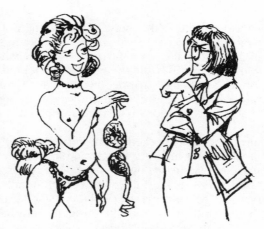

'A stripper or a headmistress'

5

Hospital

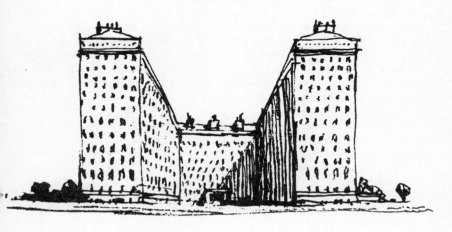

Like a conscientious parent who skips over the nasty bits in a child's favourite book and hurries on to the next page, the experts who prepare mothers for birth and motherhood gloss over the moment between delivering the baby and getting him home – the days in hospital. Increasingly, hospitals allow mothers, even first-time ones, to stay in for a shorter and shorter period after giving birth – but hospital policies still vary widely, some booting you out after twenty-four hours, others encouraging you to stay for five days.

Although the advice, help and moral support that you get in a hospital can be invaluable, no one actually *enjoys* being in hospital, even the nicest one in the world; and I'm a great believer in preparing for the worst.

Of course hospitals vary from the Victorian ones (where Sisters discourage breast-feeding, snatch the baby away to a nursery every night and most days only allow the husbands in for five minutes each evening), to the progressive ones (so liberal that the baby is left to yell by the exhausted mother's side all through the night, is discouraged from the bottle until nurses have witnessed it being glued to the breast for at least ten minutes and visitors are allowed to come in all sizes of groups at any hour of the day).

But wherever you are, you'll probably feel the same: you're uncomfortable, you're exhausted, and, most likely, you're depressed. Nearly every mother in your ward will feel at some moment inadequate, guilty about not loving the baby enough or obsessively worried about its health (although through your depressed eyes it will seem that *you* are the only one with these feelings, for such is the nature of depression). What are lightly described in most books as 'the blues' or 'the vale of tears' seem like, for anything from five minutes to six weeks, the end of the world. Some say it's another hormonal upheaval; some say it's similar to post-exam depression (after all the build-up you feel curiously deflated even though you've given birth to the best baby in the world); some say that after experiencing a feeling of being the centre of attention for nine months the mother feels let down because now the person who's getting all the curtain calls and the bunches of roses is not her, but the baby; some say that anyone who'd been carrying a huge weight around for nine months, spent, sometimes, forty-eight hours awake, involved in exhausting physical work and some pain, experienced a minor operation (for such is the episiotomy), taken drugs and then put into a ward with a lot of noise, to be woken sometimes twice a night for an hour – anyone who'd gone through all this would certainly be on the brink of depression, if not ready to Name Names into the bargain (another problem when it comes to registering the child, but more of that later).

And all of this isn't helped by mothers being given almost no warning or information about the days in hospital. Of course I'd be wrong not to mention here the joy and exhilaration from having a baby that people begin to experience in hospital ... but now I have mentioned it, let us look at the not-so joyous-and-exhilarating aspect of your week.

First there's the physical side. 'You can always tell a maternity ward,' one doctor told me, 'by the fact that it is indistinguishable from the geriatric ward except that the occupants are half the age.'

Patients in a maternity ward walk very slowly. They either shuffle like Japanese ladies in hobble skirts or they waddle like Donald Ducks, vast in their best quilted dressing-gowns – you expect them to start quacking any minute. They walk slowly because of the pain of the episiotomy – and for this use an anaesthetic spray which I mentioned before. Ask, too, for a rubber cushion with a hole in the middle, like a giant corn-plaster on which to sit in bed or at meal-times. And do take those salt-baths that the nurses will encourage you to take. 'Why?' I asked. 'Well, it's rather like curing a pig,' explained one of the nurses, alarmingly frank. 'The salt hardens the skin and makes you heal quicker.' Despite the indignity of lugging a rubber cushion around and soaking in deep, salted water for hours on end like an old chick-pea, any remedy is to be encouraged.

At the moment when your tail end is at its most painful, life isn't helped by the fact that it's very difficult to go to the loo. You will be encouraged to rise from your bed, shuffle down the ward (near-fainting is not uncommon on the way) and arrive at the loo (often engaged) only to have to sit for hours with a nurse outside shouting: 'Hurry up, or we'll have to put a catheter up you!' Peace and quiet are the best remedies; the sound of running water helps some people; best of all is a flannel soaked in very hot water held between the legs to relax the muscles – and do take a magazine to read; it'll relieve the tension.

Constipation can get very uncomfortable and the usual remedies of first, Senakot, then a suppository and finally an enema will produce results in the end.

Pain is tiring enough but exhaustion won't be helped by the arrival most days of the physiotherapist. 'Well, ladies,' announces this trim creature usually sporting a wide elastic belt to emphasize her twenty-three-inch waist, 'none of this lounging around! On your backs and *up* with the right leg . . . higher, higher, Mrs Brown, you can do better than that, get those tummy muscles firm and hard again . . . I saw you Mrs Peters! I said reach up and touch your toes not your knees. We'll soon have you looking better than before you got pregnant . . . !' I'm afraid that she is right, of course. Tedious as they may be, exercises *will* help you get your figure back.

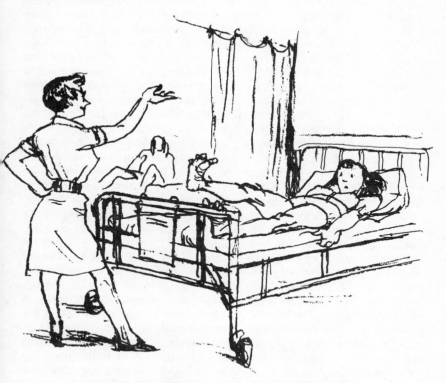

'Higher, higher, Mrs Brown, you can do better than that'

Hospital food won't exactly cheer you up, either. One friend of mine lived on Black Magic for three days until her husband sneaked her in some Marks and Spencer sandwiches.

While the hospital staff are a help, they haven't heard of sleep. It always strikes me as strange that the nurses, so keen on mothers getting their rest, seem to spend their time waking you up at 5.30 a.m., clanking iron trolleys of breakfast around, refusing to let you lie in.

Because although your baby is most likely to sleep a lot more during this week than he will at home, the demands of this new creature are also tiring. As far as these go you'll be helped if you're in an old-fashioned 'babies should be neither seen nor heard' hospital; if you find yourself in a liberal one which encourages your baby to be with you day and night, you *must* ask that it should be taken to the nursery at night unless you are in exceptionally cracking form. Few first mums forget those lonely 4.00 a.m. feeds, struggling with an awkward feeding bra in a dim reading-light, the sound of the dawn chorus drowned by interminable shrieking from the baby.

He may look strange, too, which will worry you (particularly when, as happens in some hospitals now, attention is drawn to his looks by the arrival of the hospital photo lady, who kindly snaps your baby with a giant Polaroid). His head may be covered in red blotches and marks, he may display a scalpful of weird black hair even though you and your husband may be blond (this will drop out, incidentally). In the first couple of days he'll probably not be washed and he'll be covered with dried slime; and if he moves it's only to sneeze like a cat, wave his bandy arms around, go bright red and scrunch his face up as he dirties his nappy, or sometimes to open his tiny eyes and stare strangely and unblinkingly at you like a visitor from outer space. 'Cripes, not you,' he seems to be saying.

Every day you'll trundle your cot up and down corridors to the nursery along with other mums, rather as though you're doing a weekly shop at a supermarket. Then you'll be taught how to bathe the baby, wipe the remains of his umbilical cord, clean his ears and bottom, change his nappies and put on his regimental hospital nightie. (This has such an effect of uniformity that it is not uncommon, for the first few days, for mothers to start solicitously cleaning their babies only to find after five minutes that they've got the wrong one.)

Exhaustion is topped by a social life exaggerated even by hospital standards with the whole ward yakking away from dawn till dusk about their babies' births, how wonderful/awful they feel, whether Dextrose is better than boiled water, what to do about green stools; the non-stop visits of nurses and doctors to check your breasts and your scars; the pediatricians who'll arrive to throw the baby into the air like professional pancake-makers (or so it seems to the nervous mum) to see if his reflexes are right, and the students who come to take blood samples from the baby seconds after he has finally gone to sleep. And all accompanied by the sound of yelling babies in the background. Visitors may not think it so noisy since the background buzz of small cries sounds to them only like the chirpings of crickets. To a new mother, however, all the crying sounds like a stereophonic version of the death scene in 'La Traviata' – howls of emotion from a thousand Domingos and Callases.

Less confident mothers (and most first mums fall into the 'less-confident' category) may prefer the reassuring gossip of the ward; anyone who reassures them that everything will be all right in the end, even the mad alcoholic in the end bed who already has ten children and different boyfriends to match, is welcomed. Even the ward wallies who spend their time popping down to the hospital shop for another consignment of fluffy yellow bunnies. But you may be a mother who longs for privacy – in which case it is always worth *asking* if there is a more private bed in an amenity room off the main ward. Nurses are so accustomed to patients who thrive on social ward life that it never occurs to them to offer a more secluded spot, if there is one.

Up to a point you can decide how much social life you want by vetting the visitors. Use your partner as the agent in these matters. If you don't want to be tired you should refuse *all* visitors except grandparents, who not only will long to come but will help you by reinforcing love for a baby which, from the depths of hospital gloom, can sometimes seem a difficult acquisition.

If you have to have other visitors, remember that they always stay too long. You should make it clear from the moment they arrive that you are very tired and can only spare ten minutes. They always say: 'Aren't you clever!', 'Aren't you proud!' and, 'Isn't he lovely!' These phrases are on the lines of 'How do you do?' and, 'Nice weather for the time of year' and should not be taken seriously. (I point this out because *any* remark addressed to you in this emotionally chaotic time can set up a sleepless night. I remember bursting into tears after the fourth visitor had told me how proud I must be, agonised with guilt that I didn't feel proud at all.)

Encourage your visitors to bring champagne, Badedas, bubble baths, Eau de Cologne sprays or fruit rather than flowers. By the time you leave the hospital you won't want to see another carnation or tulip in your life.

On top of all this is the insuperable task of naming your baby – you must register him no less than forty-two days after the birth. What to call the baby? Or 'it' as you will probably refer to him at this early stage, for 'it' he is until he becomes a John or an Ann. (And both these names, while they may seem dull later, now seem hopelessly fancy and ornate for this small being who doesn't appear to merit anything so grand as a sex, let alone a name.) But name him you must. Both you and your husband will have strange prejudices that prevent you calling him, say, Richard (you were once seduced by a horrible Richard), or her, Emma (he went to kindergarten with an Emma who smelt). Beware of suitable names that result in unsuitable initials (Lorna Olivia Osborne), and don't kid yourself that by giving the child seven names you give him a choice. Even Zak Horatio Barnaby Wayne John Tab Brown has no choice if all his life

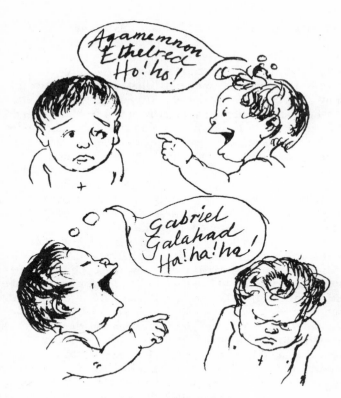

'What to call the baby?'

he's been known to his friends and relatives as Nipper.

Finally, after your time is up, you will place your baby in a carrycot, put on the baggy dress you wore when you came in, which now flaps around your thin little body like a sail on a windy day, and sheepishly carry him out of the ward to the cheers of the nurses who cry: 'See you in nine months, dear!'

Muttering: 'Not on your life!' under your breath, you hurry out of the hospital and take the baby home.

6

Home Again

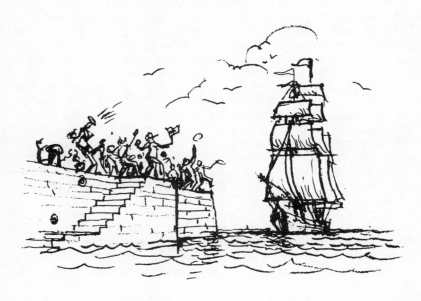

Away from the cocktail-party atmosphere of the hospital ward, life at home seems like solitary confinement in comparison, particularly if you've been working up to the birth. Your new role feels less like the beginning of a new life for yourself than the end of any life of your own at all. Even the loyal 'dad' will have beetled back to work leaving you completely on your own to look after this small person who is going to dominate your life for the next few years.

Your lonely vigils, however, are at least action-packed. The washing-machine whirs with the sound of nighties and cardigans being cleaned (at least I hope it does; no mother should be without a washing-machine); the phone seems to be always ringing just as you're in the middle of changing the baby, and life is one long chore all the way round the clock. No mother can actually remember how she did spend all that time during the first few months. All she recalls is that they were just a round of buying zinc and castor-oil ointment, reading the labels on jars of

31

sterilising liquid and dried milk, thanking people by letter for their gifts of nylon bunnies on bits of pink ribbon, trying to stop the baby crying and getting up all night to do heaven knows what but probably just sitting, anxiously wondering if the baby is still breathing, feeding him, changing him, playing with him and worrying about him.

One thing that astonished me was how demanding a baby is in the first few weeks. A mother's day will last from 7 a.m. to 11 p.m., and that's if she's exceptionally lucky. The baby may well demand feeds eight times a day rather than six – and remember that *each feed* can take up to at least an hour, what with preparing it, winding the baby, changing him, settling him and clearing up. Many baby books give a laughable 'schedule' of work for the mother that includes shopping, resting, mending and reading – but don't for one minute think that you'll be able to read so much as a headline during the first month, and don't feel the least bit guilty if you can't either. Eight hours a day may well be spent just feeding him, anyway, so you'll barely have time even to get dressed during the day. The nights are nearly always bad since he may well prefer to sleep from seven in the evening until one in the morning when he wakes, rather than from midnight until six in the morning (which is when you're told he will sleep). The first few days must be spent in weaning him away from the hospital routine – when you fitted your life completely into his – into a home routine when you try your hardest to get him to fit into *your* schedule.

Since you'll be very lucky if you get so much as six hours sleep a night (and that usually in three-hour bursts) it's essential at this time to make things as easy as possible for yourself, particularly remembering that you've only just recovered from something as exhausting as a major operation and are working flat out, sometimes twenty hours a day, seven days a week.

It's really too easy, if you're not properly prepared, to begin to loathe your child during these days – mainly because you wouldn't be feeling so exhausted or have so much to do and have so little time to do it in, if it weren't for him. But a baby *is* really very companionable; if you were married to a millionaire and had a staff of servants running around doing the chores there's no doubt that far from finding the first weeks a chore you'd spend them in a state of euphoria. So it's very important to gear your life to make the drudgery less – and be able to give yourself the time to make the most of your baby.

To make life possible requires preparation and thought. First, before you even return home from hospital, your partner should have prepared the house for a six-week siege and have bought up the maximum of supplies – tins of all description, tons of washing powder, sacks of potatoes, loo paper, cans of beer – in fact as much of everything that will save you having to venture to the shops for about six weeks. And ensure that if you *do* have to go out, you won't have to carry anything very heavy back home. Any friends who ring asking what kind of present you would like should be told to drop round with a casserole for your supper – and to leave you immediately to eat in peace.

Then there's the housework. I found those strictures to leave the housework alone practically impossible because a messy, dirty house always depresses me – and I did feel better when I'd done the cleaning, however exhausted I felt. The only answer is to reduce your living space. Move into the bedroom and live in it like a bedsitter. Drag in the television, deck the place up with all those hospital flowers (that you must bring home with you – don't leave them in gratitude to the nurses who would anyway prefer a bottle of champagne), give up all ideas of dressing and wear your prettiest night clothes and dressing-gown all day.

If you can afford it, get some help. Monthly nurses are very expensive, and have a tendency to spend all their time looking after the baby while you hike to the shops and clean the kitchen floor. It might be better to spend the money, anyway, on a temporary daily, particularly a nice one who has kids of her own and would be a willing psychological help while she was around. If you can't afford paid help, accept the help of a mother or mother-in-law, but only if you're absolutely sure you'll be able to get by without rows. I was lucky with mine, but many mothers-in-law make too much fuss about the baby, irritate you with old-fashioned notions of feeding routines and fresh air, and spend most of their time worrying about whether the baby is too hot or too cold. None of these concerns are unimportant, of course, but with better medical care these days more attention is paid to the baby's emotional rather than physical welfare.

If you're desperate for moral support, the health visitor can be a good source. She comes within the week of your return from hospital (and for many weeks more if you wish) and usually sits with kindly eyes, asking if you have any problems. She may be an old grey-haired spinster with endless good advice or a mother of three with no idea of what you feel. Mine was a childless woman who kept asking me if I thought she should adopt. Every time she came I felt like smashing a frying pan over her head. How on earth should I know, for heavens sake? I should have asked for a different health visitor – it's quite possible to do this – because, like most mothers, I had a list of problems that I would reel off in a panic to anyone who would listen.

'But sex is agony, I'll never be able to make love again . . .' (Don't worry, dear, it's very common.) 'But he cries all the time!' (Oh, the rascal, you've either got a good baby or One of Them. You've got One of Them.) 'He wakes eight times a night!' (Some mothers' babies only sleep for two hours a night, dear; think yourself lucky.) 'But I can't cope!' (Your concern shows what a good mother you are. Don't worry.)

You'll need every bit of help you can get because during this period you'll be super-sensitive to anything said by anyone in authority. The doctor only has to have something in his eye when listening to the baby's heart and the resulting faint puckering of pain over his brow as he blinks will make you worry for days that the baby is going to die next week. A nurse only has to say: 'Why not give him a little bit of cereal in his feed at night to see if that will help him sleep?' and this gets translated, in the long, lonely hours of brooding, into thinking that she means that he's a most peculiar baby to wake so often and that she's very worried about him indeed. This is no moment to keep a stiff upper lip. Show your tearful reactions at once, to avoid a week of sleepless nights.

And if any little helpful hint can make you cry for days, a tiny bit of helpful criticism can unhinge you completely. The mother-in-law who starts any sentence to the new mother with: 'Why don't you . . .' or, 'Are you sure he doesn't need a . . .' immediately places herself in danger of being slipped large quantities of sterilising fluid in her next cup of coffee, being strangled with a nappy liner or mangled by the wheels of a heavy pram.

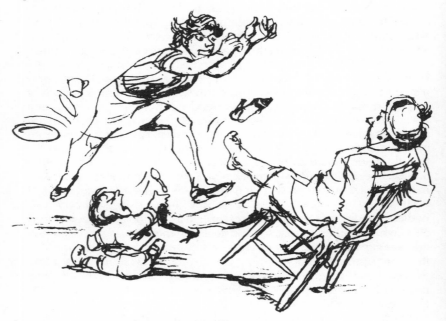

'Are you sure he doesn't need a . . .'

'Isn't he a bit cold?' is a remark that can send the new mother into a rage – it implies she's freezing the baby to death through criminal negligence. When an aunt of mine picked the baby's dummy from the floor and proceeded to wash it before handing it back to him she wasn't asked back to my house for nine months. My floor? Dirty? How *dare* she?

It may well be that you are anyway suffering from post-natal depression, something very different to those baby blues you probably went through in hospital. Post-natal depression is not at all like ordinary depression, which is why so many mothers don't spot they're suffering from it. It usually takes the form of acute anxiety, guilt, feelings of total inadequacy and a general conviction that as a mother you are about as useful to your baby as a gerbil. The moment you start feeling you're a total fraud and completley useless is the moment to consult your doctor because action taken at an early stage can prevent a lot of misery later.

There are quite a few degrees of post-natal depression, from mild to acute. The mild may take the form of thinking you dislike your new baby, knowing (irrationally of course) that you are a hopeless mother, bursting into tears at the slightest thing and often becoming obsessed with your baby's health. Some mothers have panic attacks and find going out to the shops an insuperable task.

The more severe form of post-natal depression is the same only much, much worse. You feel you don't love your baby; you may think about putting him into care so he can have a better life (yes, that's how warped one's mind can get); you may have fantasies about harming your baby which frighten you – even though it's extremely unlikely you would ever actually do anything to hurt him, even if you think you might. Everything seems black. Your doctor really can help you, probably with anti-depressants which are worth taking to tide you through a horrible patch that will, eventually, disappear.

Puerperal psychosis is the *creme de la creme* of post-natal depression and luckily it only occurs in two out of every thousand mothers. In this case the mother has delusions and completely loses touch with reality. Usually this involves having to go to hospital for treatment, but happily this treatment is nearly always extremely effective and within weeks the mother is back to her old self.

Obviously it helps if during this time the families can rally round in a way that's constructive and doesn't make the problem even worse. And although I've mentioned some appalling relations, they're not all maddening. And visits from relations serve an important purpose – they turn you from a part of a couple with a baby into part of a family. A partner who might have been looked on as a mere appendage to yourself that has had to be put up with by your relations is now drawn into your own family circle because he exists in this new person, their grandchild. Similarly, by having a baby you'll be drawn into *his* family in a way that even getting married can never quite do. A baby makes an almost chemical change in you and your relationships.

Close relatives, far relatives, relatives no one ever knew existed – all these move in during the first week back home to peer at this new addition to the family, all determined to claim him as more like their side of the family than the other's. Certainly, as Granny Brown and Granny Smith meet by accident over tea, the conversation runs on one track.

'He's got the Smith eyes exactly.'

'Oh, but you know all baby's eyes are blue when they're born. I can tell they're going to change. I think they'll be dark – like us Browns.'

35

'Well, he's certainly very long.' (Babies are always long, not tall since they can't stand up; however, they are not wide nor are they fat – they're 'bonny'.) 'He's going to be a big boy like his father.'

'Perhaps,' concedes Granny Smith, 'but there's no doubt he's got the Smith nose.'

'He most certainly has!' replies Granny Brown, acidly.

As you can see from the above it's far better from your point of view to keep families apart during the first few weeks. The sight of two new grannies haggling and tussling over your baby's features is a strain.

The best contribution from relatives, however, is a reassuring jargon. (Baby-sitting and help with the housework is welcome, but watch out that the grannies don't stake too much of a claim to the household while they fetch and carry; you might regret it later.) If you've given birth to some slothful oaf who does nothing but snooze all day and has to be woken for his feeds, appears to be permanently stoned, opens his eyes only occasionally and feebly to give a half-hearted smile before sinking back into torpor, then the relatives will exclaim that he is a 'contented' baby.

'What a lovely child, he's so content!' they say soothingly, digging him rather too hard in the ribs to get a smile out of him. 'Yes he really is' (as he doesn't bat an eyelid), 'he's a contented little soul.'

If, on the other hand, you have given birth to a fiend in baby shape, a character who howls day and night, whose face is always contorted into a blue-red blur of rage, who kicks and screams, bites and flies into

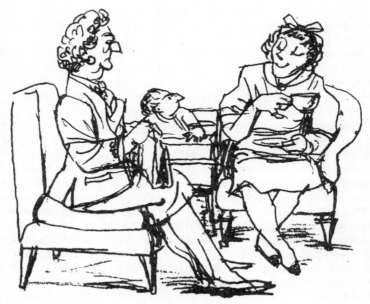

'There's no doubt he's got the Smith nose'

paroxysms if anyone so much as whispers on the rare occasions he sleeps, then he is deemed an 'alert' baby.

'Oh, he's an intelligent one, he's so alert, isn't he?' the relatives say, or rather shout, over his screams. 'He'll go far. Isn't he alert?'

You'll find, too, that it's not only relations who hover around. Everyone you ever knew wants to visit you, from the wife of the tobacconist on the corner to long-lost school-friends who, seeing an announcement in the papers, suddenly turn up to see the baby. With such visitors it's not so much a case of 'Now I know who my real friends are'; rather, 'Now I know which of my friends like babies.' While comparative strangers are clamouring at the door to visit you, old, close, single men friends may scamper off to the country or find they're too busy even to send a card; close, childless women friends are embarrassed to find your life has taken this new twist at last and feel you different and disloyal in the same way as your single girlfriends felt when you settled down with your partner.

And if you live in a town, most likely your doorbell won't stop ringing. Lonely teenagers come to call, anxious to take the baby for walks, or just come in and tickle him under the chin.

One benefit of visitors is the fact that they will all (or should all) come bearing gifts. Life becomes one long round of opening parcels containing outsize yellow sleepsuits, apparently useless V-necked jerseys, miniscule leather baby-shoes that he'll never wear, weird cubes of sanded wood with bells inside and a lot of other stuff that may well strike you, initially, as junk. Whatever you do, don't be too sniffy about these contributions which, you will find to your amazement later, will nearly all prove to be useful.

Someone kind and thoughtful will undoubtedly provide a mobile, for which, as you attempt to rig it up, you will curse them. A cardboard circus-master, two prancing horses, three sealions balancing red balls on their noses and an elephant, all suspended by an invisible thread should, in theory be twirling and jiggling round the baby's head giving him something stimulating to look at. But to get it up? Evenings of ingenious work must be spent balancing chairs on tables at angles with books under a couple of the legs so that the mobile hangs exactly over his face. It's only after all this sweat when your baby lies silently entranced that you'll realise that a mobile is perhaps the most sensible and useful present of all. A mobile is, after all, nothing but a very early form of television.

The reason you're so choosy about the gifts you receive is simply because you, like most new mothers, are driven by an urge towards perfection. And, it must be said, most of it is time wasted. It's only three cheque books later that you catch on that most of those supplies of cot-sheets, baby soaps, cotton-wool balls, safety-glass film, cotton buds, special soap flakes and baby baths are just so much conspicuous consumption.

As for the gadgets, a friend of mine found her sitting-room converted into a kind of dwarf's gym, with playpens, baby-bouncers, portable seats, high-chairs, dolphin crawlers, baby-walkers and bouncing cradles. It's possible, with help from friends lending a minimum of equipment and conscientious sifting through the small ads in tobacconists' windows, to obtain everything a new-born baby needs for less than £50. It's also possible to turn your house into a nightmare of trusses hanging from doors, folding wheels in corridors and brand-new cooker guards for over £350.

Guard not only against this frantic desire to give the baby the best but also try to get a grip on your inevitable obsession with your baby's health. Most mothers experience this; if not, a few visits to the clinic to weigh the baby will soon get you in the way of it.

Watch out, too, for the time when your friendly GP will give the baby a reflex test – a series of horrible sensations to test his reactions.

She will clap her hands loudly on either side of his head, hold him up hanging on to her finger and shine a torch in his eyes. There is, of course, no winning at this game. If he doesn't respond your doctor will start worrying. If he reacts, it usually means he howls for the rest of the morning – proof that he's sensitive. And do remember that unless your baby loses some weight or gains only a minute fraction of what he should, there is *no need* to worry about fattening him up if you're offering him adequate food. Don't hang about waiting for him to coo with pleasure (and thus open his mouth) in order to plunge a giant spoonful of gooey cereal down him. It's more likely to give him problems with food for life than help him gain weight.

At some point, if you're so inclined, you'll think about a christening – which is a great excuse for a party, even if you're not so concerned with the godly aspects of it as you might be.

A christening should be a hugely jolly and happy occasion with the baby dressed in a proper christening dress (particularly charming if he happens to be a boy) which can usually be begged or borrowed from a friend; a small party afterwards can deal with a lot of visits that might be too exhausting on their own.

The baby must have no fewer than three godparents (but remember you and your partner can be godparents if you're pushed) and, apart from promising to see the child is brought up to follow Christ, there is nothing a godparent has to do. But who to pick? It's tempting, of course, to choose a childless, confirmed bachelor or spinster, who is unlikely ever to produce, with a vast fortune waiting to be left to your baby. A godparent, however, is not just an easy touch.

It's worth thinking about making a relation a godparent, to give him or her a special relationship with the child; and also try to include someone middle-aged. It's no good giving your child a sexy young air hostess as a godparent, who is planning on emigrating to Australia to set up a family. A close friend who's just had a baby might be a good choice in the long term, too (particularly if you can be a godparent to her child as well) as she's in a good position to understand all your child's problems at every stage in it's life.

In these first few weeks of bringing the baby home you'll be exhausted, fraught and anxious. It's quite possible that sex may be a problem. And if you've had an episiotomy *and* you're exhausted from being up all night with the baby, small wonder you feel fairly uninterested. On top of all this, you may feel that sex has achieved its purpose for the time being and you're simply uninterested in even thinking about reproduction for the moment. Look where it got you, after all! Speaking personally, I didn't think the six weeks after the birth, after which most doctors think you might be coming round to the idea again, was long enough, and research has shown that most women don't find sexual feelings returning until ten to twelve weeks after the birth. If your partner were helping you as much as he should be, he would probably be far too tired even to get to work on time, let alone thinking of sex. If you can't face it after two months and if it's causing your partner all kinds of agonies, then obviously the only decent thing you can do is to visit your doctor to show, at least, that you are considering the problem.

If you're breast-feeding, hormonal changes may well be responsible for making you feel less sexy (though do remember that it's only if you're breast-feeding every two hours that it works as a contraception; anything less than that and you ought to be using birth-control unless you want another baby straight away, and if you do you must be mad). If the baby wakes a lot at night you may be too exhausted for sex. Or you may simply have no time at all for it. Considering your mind is a whirring mass of questions – is he hungry, is he ill, does he need changing, are you a good mum or not, is he breathing? – there's often just no time to think of sex. Sometimes an episiotomy scar may make sex a bit on the ouchy side (KY jelly bought at a chemist can make sex a bit more comfortable); or it could be that now you've produced a baby your body just shuts down on the idea of further reproduction for a short while. 'Now I've delivered a baby I don't need to worry about any more sex for the moment, thank you,' it seems to be saying.

However, quite often you've just got out of the habit, and usually, after you've managed to make love two or three times, you slip back into the old ways. It's rather like jumping into a cold swimming-pool. Agony for a few minutes but lovely once you're in. Well, fairly lovely.

On top of all this, feelings will be exaggerated out of all proportion. The loneliness, the tied-down feelings, the pathetic little weeps of pleasure ('But they're so sweet!' I kept sobbing as my husband asked why I was weeping over ironing my baby's tiny nightdresses), the fury that can burst out any minute even when just kept waiting a few minutes in a shop – this is what is most memorable about the first stage of motherhood. And there is little to be said in conclusion except what everyone will tell you (and, if you are like me and most new mothers, you simply won't believe it) – it will all be over much too soon. That little face you've been stuffing with mashed bananas all too quickly sprouts a beard; the little piping voice that lisps 'Mummy' will change into a deep, drawling buzz in what seems like a matter of months when you look back on it – and those tiny pink-frocked companions who used to come to tea and be helped onto the loo, appear stiff with eye-make-up and dressed head-to-toe in black in the shape of glamorous girlfriends barely before you've folded the last nappy and put it away.

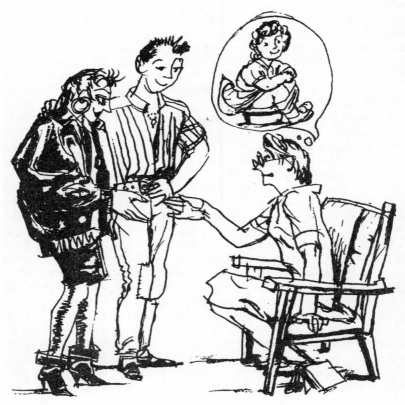

7

Motherhood

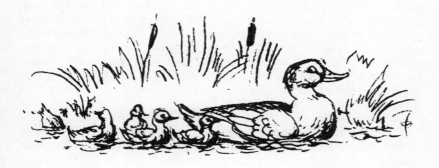

We all want to be Good Mothers. We're haunted by the fear that when the baby is grown up, he will be spending fifty minutes a day on an analyst's couch, revealing how perfectly ghastly we were during his early years. We hope desperately that he will have a memory of a mother who was *not* panic stricken, driven to battering, over-protective or useless.

And yet during the first few weeks, while other mothers seem to be able to cope perfectly well, you'll most likely find yourself completely at sea. Everywhere you go you'll see these capable matrons in the street, wheeling prams laden with toddlers sitting on seats above sleeping babies while still more children frisk behind with teddies and ice-creams.

You, on the other hand, can barely manoeuvre the pram out of the door and find it so difficult to manage anything but looking after the baby that it's a sign of a really good and productive day when you proudly tell your partner when he returns from work and asks what you've been up to: 'I had lunch!'

One way of trying to cope is to peruse every baby book in sight and spend your days consulting the doctor at the clinic. But while a baby book helps by telling you what you can do to help the baby, it will never tell you enough about what to expect to feel as a *mother* and what you can do to help your faltering steps into motherhood itself.

No one slips into motherhood straight away. It takes about two years to begin to feel in charge of the situation. And one of the first problems facing the new mother is that although birth separates her and her baby physically, emotional separation is slow. To begin with you'll be very confused about where you start and he begins. One moment the baby may seem like a new person in his own right; another, he will seem like one of your amputated limbs, wriggling away independently in a carrycot and yet still part of you. It's difficult to tell who's crying or laughing, him or you.

This feeling of union is what prompts the disconcerting theory that all upsets in a baby are caused by you, the mother. If he won't feed properly, goes one theory, then it's your fault. If he screams in the night, then it's your fault. Confusingly, there's an opposite theory that all the upsets are caused by the baby rather than the other way round. Hence babies who won't eat *make you* sick with worry – rather than your worry causing them not to eat. Clearly there is some middle way between both very plausible theories – and finding out exactly where it is is the first hard lesson in the art of motherhood.

This difficult task isn't made easier by the fact that your baby is, surprisingly, born with a personality. To non-baby-owners he is a mere blob; but he already possesses a vociferous character all of his own, which you, obviously, have very little knowledge of as yet. And *he*, on his side, has very little idea of what you are like either (except perhaps for the odd noise from a rumbling stomach, a whiff of nicotine or a heavy bump that he would certainly notice inside the womb). The first few weeks involve getting to know each other. What kind of a mother has he got himself landed with? Does he like being sung to or talked to? Is he placid or active?

Some kind of structure is essential to stop yourself being a complete slave to his whims, or him being a complete slave to yours. And yet it's important not to let the routine dominate both of you, i.e., he yells his head off at four o'clock while waiting for his six o'clock feed; or you are obliged to miss half an hour of a riveting television programme just so you can wake him up to feed him at ten o'clock on the dot. *That* way, one or other is being denied any existence at all, which is, in the long run, detrimental to your relationship.

Two common traps, uncomfortable with your new role and feeling unable to cope, are to become either 'the best mum in the world' or the 'vegetable'.

Just because everyone else assumes that because you're a mother you're an instant old hand, deft with a nappy pin, skilful at feeding and 'good' with children, you don't have to live up to their ideals. I always remember when someone soothed my baby in front of me, saying: 'Don't worry, mummy's here!', I turned, involuntarily expecting to find a stout, reassuring, aproned matron behind me. I couldn't really believe that it was *me* who was the mummy. Feelings of such inadequacy often lead to the new mother over-compensating by a zealous dedication to mother-hood and an ambition to be 'the best mum in the world' (a figure popular with those who write in for record requests on the radio). The 'best mum in the world' is an impossible ideal. This mythical creature bakes her own bread, has a comfortable lap, large bosom and a store of little cooing noises designed to soothe and comfort. Her growing baby has lunch at twelve, a nap after lunch and sleeps through the night.

One way of beating this fantasy is to pick a 'best mum in the world' (and most of us have some friend we enviously regard as perfect in every way) and confront her. When I finally plucked up courage to examine my own particular 'best mum' I found that in practice her baby didn't go to bed until nine, and when he woke at ten (after the best dad in the world had been rocking him for half an hour to get him off to sleep) his delighted parents brought him down to show him off and stuffed him with bits of sausage until midnight, when he was promptly sick.

The other danger is to turn into a cabbage. You'll have been warned that you'll turn into a vegetable after giving birth, with nothing to talk of except feeds and nappies, but no one warns you how unpleasant are the side-effects of actually *being* that vegetable.

Within a few weeks of getting home you're convinced that your life as you knew it is over, you'll never see any glittering shops again, your days are forever going to be one deadly round of sitting in a house doing nothing or wheeling the baby to the park, staring at him in the sandpit, cramming strained gooseberries down his throat and changing his nappies. As you catch a reflection of yourself in the shop windows, wheeling that hideous pram or clinging grimly to the bar of a pushchair, it's hard not to feel that no one will ever fancy you again, that your days as an attractive, wanted young woman are over and that you have turned overnight into a slaggy old bag in clumsy sandals, branded by everyone as 'just a housewife'. There'll probably be a moment when it all comes home to you when some bright, good-looking bloke with whom you've always enjoyed a mildly flirtatious, winking relationship, will clap you on the back and say in a jovial voice: 'Well, how's mum?' And in a moment you'll be cast down, feeling old and plump and baggy and good for nothing except straining carrots and wiping bottoms.

With your life circumscribed by the baby, nappy bucket and food strainer, you'll worry, with reason, about your conversation going downhill as well – which it probably will. For the health visitor and baby books and elderly relations will encourage you to 'talk to your baby'. But about what? The state of the Labour Party? The plight of Soviet dissidents? The horrors of plutonium waste? No. You're inevitably reduced to talking rubbish.

'See the pretty colours!' 'Oooh, what a burp!' 'Look at the ducks – quack, quack!' Eighty per cent of the time you'll be so involved with the baby that this simply won't seem like drivel to you (and actually I found talking this drivel a great release after a lifetime of bright adult chit-chat

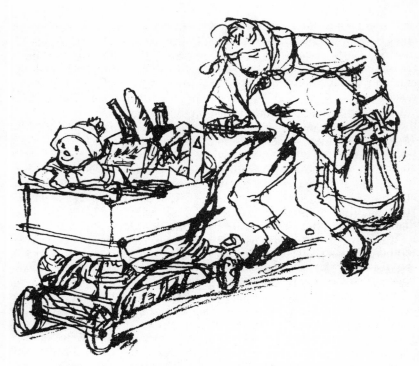

'It's hard not to feel that no one will ever fancy you again'

on topics of the day). But *do* remember that it does sound like drivel to other people. And if you're alone all day with the baby, it becomes a habit. It's not unknown to make an effort, throw a dinner party and spend the whole evening muttering: 'Oooh, what a nasty little bone, we must pick that out . . . will you have some more? . . . a-a-ah, come on, have a little try, just for me . . . why! I can hear a lovely fire engine in the distance, a lovely red fire engine, *red, red, red* . . . yes, just like that strawberry mousse . . .'

You may well start calling everyone 'we'. While it's one thing to say to the baby: 'Let's have our bath' – quite a normal thing to say to someone who has only a month or so back stopped being part of your body, someone, indeed, you literally have been having a bath with for nine months – it's quite a different matter to hand your guest a drink saying: 'Here's our gin and tonickins!'

It's at this stage of vegetoid frumpery that you must call a halt. Park the baby with a friend for the day, whizz into town, get your hair done and buy a new dress (and *don't* be tempted to pop into the nearest Mothercare; I remember making a momentous trip to buy a smashing new party dress and returning with three Babygros and a little woolly hat). After pregnancy your hair never looks at its best and it's usually high time it got some attention. Plan a few 'baby-swaps' with other mothers and get at least a couple of afternoons off a week to go to a gallery, see a movie, do the garden or just read a book by yourself. This might even be the moment to try to get a part-time job; certainly you must make an effort to get out and about more and force your life into perspective vis-à-vis the outside world.

Of course you *can* escape from the tedium of being cooped up with the baby by visiting other mothers. Other mothers are a mixed blessing. They will ask you over to tea (a meal that since the baby was born has become a major feature of the day) and they'll gossip with you for hours about your favourite topic – babies. Women you may have found deadly in your pre-baby days suddenly star as mines of information, sympathy and good humour when you've got a baby in common. The danger is that you'll use other mums as a way of making your life more tolerable, rather than giving yourself the necessary breaks from your baby. And of course it's true that a mother who chats all day over coffee and biscuits with other mothers often actually pays less attention to the baby in the long run than the mother who spends half a day at work and the other half concentrating on the baby full-time.

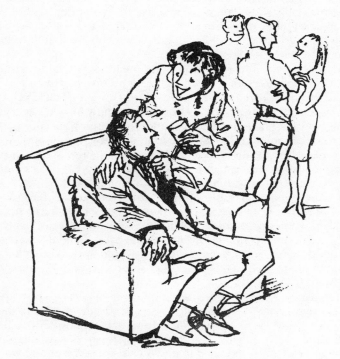

'Here's our gin and tonickins!'

Other mothers usually come in two varieties. Either they live a full, chaotic life, making mobiles out of old yoghurt cartons and weaving their own nappies, living happily in filth and squalor ('I always believe in letting the house go if you've got a baby!' they say, merrily looking at you with a conspiratorially maternal grin through a haze of dust as they hitch up their collapsing tights. 'After all, they're only young once!')

Or they're paragons of neatness, immaculate in matching jerseys and cardigans under sponge-clean aprons, with kitchen rolls at the ready to wipe the faintest trace of food from the baby's face, able to stuff red peppers with truffles and garlic paté in kitchens already wired up with safety gadgets in anticipation of the toddler stage and still happy to produce gins and tonics with slices of lemon and ice every evening at six with no more than a little help. (They, of course, in their turn, will be putting you into one of these categories, too.)

It's through these other mothers that you'll be introduced to the jargon of motherhood. 'He sleeps through' doesn't mean he goes to bed in a tunnel with his head sticking out at one end and his feet another; it means he sleeps without waking at night. 'Soon he'll be quite a handful' doesn't mean 'a handful'; it means *both* hands full. 'He's into everything' doesn't mean pottery and yoga and basket-weaving but cupboards full of bleach and burning oil-stoves. 'Putting him down' isn't a euphemism for killing him painlessly; it means putting him to bed. 'He's gone off' doesn't mean he's starting growing mould like old cheese or suddenly made his escape; it means he's gone to sleep.

As well as a new culture, motherhood means a new family structure. You're no longer just someone's daughter; your own mother is no longer just your mummy. *You* are a mummy. *She* is a granny. It may be hard for you to cope with being a mummy but your mummy turned into a granny is stranger by far. And not only is your mother a granny but your partner's mother is a granny too. Not to mention your stepmother and, in these days of easy divorce, his stepmother as well, all eager to get in on the granny act. There can't be four people called granny. (There are only two legitimate ones anyway, and they have to fight it out between themselves.) And at least a couple of these grandparents will have decided already what they want to be called whether you or he like it or not. I was astonished when one of these, a woman I regarded as reasonably sane, announced: 'Come to Tanma, darling!' to the baby. Tanma! Next thing I'd hear would be that one of the grandfathers would want to be called Gaga. And sure enough – 'No, that's your Gaga over there,' said 'Tanma'. '*This* is your Tanma!'

You're likely to see more of grandmothers than before – because they will, of course, want to see the baby – so just resign yourself to this and take advantage of the rest you'll get at their houses because they'll be so busy fussing over the baby. Use them shamelessly as babysitters when you do go out, and remember that two Christmases running with one grannie will send the other one spare with jealousy. Stick to Christmases

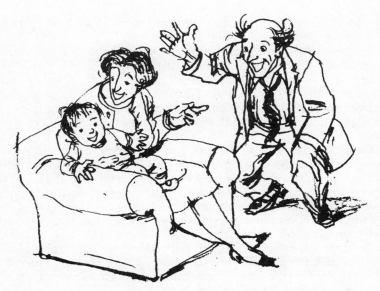

'No, that's your Gaga over there'

at home from the start to avoid trouble later on.

You'll be going out, actually, much less than you used to, of course. Not just because you're so tired but because the ties of motherhood do allow you to take liberties with your social life. A visit to hospital to cheer up a delirious acquaintance must be dismissed on the grounds that 'it's such a pity the hospital won't allow babies in'. 'So sorry we can't come to hear you play the oboe in the church hall,' you must say to that dismal music student of a cousin, 'but we can't get a sitter.' And, 'I'd love to come on a walking tour through the Pennines,' you must say to your partner as he longingly eyes his pair of hob-nailed boots, 'But what about him . . . the little one? I think it would be much nicer for him to go to a nice little rented cottage in the country . . .'

At the end of the day motherhood really means worry. Are you doing right? Are you spoiling the baby? Are you traumatising him? If he finds you in bed with daddy will he be jealous? If daddy finds him in bed with you, will his daddy be jealous? If he comes into your bed at all will he still be in your bed when he's sixteen? If you give him sweets now will his teeth rot? Should you let him cry or run to him at every whimper? If you shout at him will he be terrified? If you don't shout at him, will he be repressed?

In the middle of this whirlwind of fears and questions keep hold of two facts. First: it's not what you do, it's how you do it. Mothers all over the world bring their children up very differently; some feed them one thing, some feed them another; some breast-feed until the children are four years old; others never breast-feed them; some wrap them up tightly; some leave them free.

And secondly, babies are very different to each other. A friend of mine, worried about the effect she appeared to be having on her first child, who was a little monster, felt relief from guilt only when she produced another, a complete angel, and so different from the first that she had to realise that his problems weren't all of her own making. Some babies are difficult and some aren't. And the difficult ones are all difficult in different ways.

Guilt, indeed, plays an important part in motherhood and perhaps simply acknowledging that from now on you're going to spend at least half to three-quarters of your life feeling needlessly guilty is a better way of coping with it than trying not to feel guilty, something that I've never found possible. I first felt guilty about not having 'bonded' properly with my son. I was never quite sure what bonding was, except that it sounded like something to do with Evostik, until I read a hair-raising article that assured me that if I hadn't properly bonded with my baby from birth – in other words, been in close contact with him for the first twenty-four hours or so of his life – then our relationship, not to mention his future, was doomed. It so happened that in my case, due to a major hospital botch-up in the episiotomy department which involved an operation the day following the birth, bonding simply wasn't possible. It was only years of guilt later that I read that the bonding theory has completely gone up the spout in some circles and that there was no need to worry about it at all.

Next on my list of guilty worries was maternal instinct. What exactly was it? It was like a bar of soap; just as I thought I'd got near to getting the hang of it, it slipped out of my grasp. Although others all around me assured that if anyone had maternal instinct, I was blessed with sackfuls, I never felt quite easy with the term. It was something about that word 'instinct', as if the ability to change nappies and sing lullabies should be embedded in ones genes. It never quite felt like that.

The guilt was compounded, as it always is, by the fact that because I had these worries, I was convinced, by reading endless loopy baby books, that these inner doubts would convey themselves to my baby and that he would grow up a raving neurotic, a deeply unhappy young man who would probably commit suicide at thirteen because of some deep-rooted misery that I had instilled in him when he was a tiny baby. Needless to say he still seems full of beans at fifteen, but I only have to see the odd shadow pass over his face and I am, ridiculously, convinced that it's due to something dreadful I thought or did that he picked up in his past – when almost certainly it's simply his maths prep that's to blame. I mention all this only in order to reassure those of you who feel the same as I did that these feelings are not only common, they are rife – and also ridiculous.

But I suspect that motherhood is only a real problem for us when it's new and difficult. It is only the mothers of a first child who moan about washing nappies and being cut off from their friends. It's not the nappy-washing and the pram-pushing in itself which is so exhausting, but the fact that new mothers get into a tizz about them. And after one child you're an old pro, talking casually about 'the kids', never at a loss as to what to do on a wet Sunday, never panicking at the slightest whimper or snuffle. When you've gone through it once, it must seem so simple that you can't imagine what the fuss was about.

8

Crying

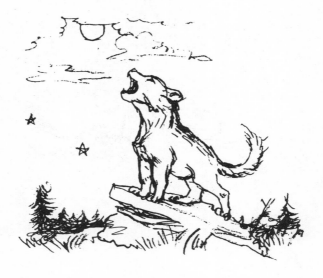

Just talking about their babies' crying reduces most mothers to tears. A crying baby is exhausting; a crying baby grates on your nerves and deprives you of sleep; a crying baby would extract more secrets from spies than any number of cigarettes stubbed out on their feet.

Every mother, especially an emotionally vulnerable first mother of just a few months, would agree that there's something about the sound of their own baby crying that touches the deepest nerves – and a mere whimper in the night that leaves your partner snoring loudly may well find you sitting bolt up in bed with your hair standing on end, panicking about what on earth is wrong with him.

The great trick is to know where to draw the line between leaving him to cry and paying attention to him. There *are* mothers who blithely leave their babies to yell themselves to sleep in darkened rooms alone; there *are* also mothers who race to the cot with nappies, cuddles and drinks of water every time the baby so much as squeaks.

But the aim of both is to shut the child up. The mum who leaves the

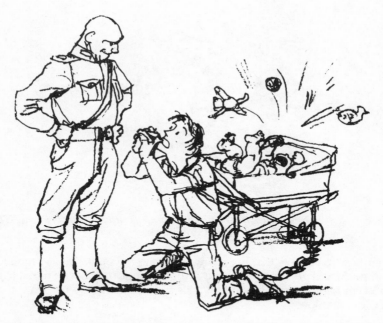

'A crying baby would extract more secrets from spies than any number of cigarettes stubbed out on their feet'

baby to cry is planning in the long term, hoping that the baby will cotton on to the fact that crying will get it nowhere (but this theory might be dangerous if the child simply gets the impression that nobody cares about it at all). The mum who springs into action at the first whimper believes that satisfying the child's needs will make him feel secure, and he'll cry less in the future (but this theory might make him feel that crying is *too* important and that anger and misery are powerful and dangerous emotions).

It is clearly not the end of the world to let the baby have a good bawl from time to time, as long as you are close by and sympathetic (not to exercise his lungs, as some old people still contend, but to let him experience his rage and fear to the full in security with no earth-shattering results). But it's the relaxed mother who's confident that she loves the child and can give a laugh, albeit slightly resentful, when he starts up, who can leave him to cry the most successfully. More common is the mum who finds crying brings *her* down and eventually leaves the baby to yell because she has given up, she's fed up and she can't stand another harrowing minute. If the baby feels he's being left to cry as some kind of punishment, obviously he'll only cry harder and feel let down and rejected.

But say you're a mum who believes in giving the baby attention, or just

51

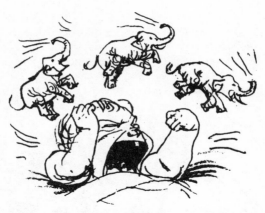

'If the baby feels he's being left to cry as some kind of punishment, obviously he'll only cry harder'

a mum who realises that his crying has gone on a little bit too long for comfort? (And personally I'm one of those frantic mums who find it hard to let any baby cry for a second.) What's wrong with him? What can you do to calm him down?

Food

He might be hungry, and nine times out of ten a feed will calm him down. He will obviously cry more if you have a rigid feeding time-table and don't allow him snacks in between. A few sips of sterilised water might also help. I myself can't think of anything less likely to stop me crying than a few sips of sterilised water, but as yet babies have no experience of anything as exciting as a Bloody Mary and seem to welcome it.

Light

Even at this tender age babies can be frightened of the dark. And how would *you* like to be placed in a box in a strange room, unable to move, with no light at all? A low light, or the light from the landing, can be soothing.

Loneliness and fear

Arguably, the confident mum is less likely to produce a baby full of loneliness and fear; and a mum who is super-sensitive might well pass her anxiety on to the baby. But if you feel he is anxious on his own, and a confident manner will not reassure him, then don't hesitate to bring him into your bed. It's *much* easier to feed him if you have him in bed in the first weeks, anyway. If you're breast-feeding you hardly have to wake up at all, but unless you go to bed dead drunk there's virtually no danger of your squashing him or of him rolling out. I *know* that you – and, more likely, your partner – will be fearful that he will still be in there when he is sixteen and bringing his girlfriends back, but he won't. At three or four anyway he will most likely want his own grown-up bed and it will be all you can do to lure him in for a cuddle in the mornings.

Discomfort

Perhaps your baby doesn't like sleeping on his back/tummy/side. Just as it's crucially important for you to be able to find a comfortable position when you sleep, so it's important for the baby. Maybe he wants more blankets, fewer blankets, or perhaps you should open or close the window.

Drugs

Desperate mothers (and not-so-desperate ones) have all resorted to going to their doctor and wheedling some elixir out of him that will help make the baby sleep at night. Some mums, at the end of their tethers, have even slipped the children a nip of sherry (a big mistake – gripe water is quite alcoholic enough containing, as it does, 4.4% alcohol); most mums have tried to introduce a tiny bit of solid food into their babies' diet at supper-time so that the babies will fall back, replete, like fat old businessmen after an expense-account lunch. (I don't recommend the sherry; and I must say that none of these cures worked for my baby. A spoonful of Farex or a dose of sleep-inducing medication against a crying baby is like setting a flea against a tiger.)

Teeth

The first tooth arrives somewhere around the sixth month, but, from the age of nought to two, much crying is put down to teething. Actually, some cultures don't acknowledge teething as a problem at all and medically it's a fairly dubious diagnosis of misery. But anyway, most babies are soothed by rusks, bits of toast, teething rings or teething jelly rubbed on the gums.

Nappies

There was a research project that involved taking a hundred screaming babies with dirty nappies, changing fifty of them into fresh nappies, and fifty of them back into their own old, dirty nappies – and they all stopped crying. It could be a dirty or wet nappy that's making the baby cry – but what he needs, often, is the attention, handling and fuss that nappy-changing gives him.

Pacifiers

However ugly you may think your beautiful baby's face looks covered with a round disc of plastic, there's no doubt that a dummy is usually a winner. He may look awful, but he sounds great – completely silent.

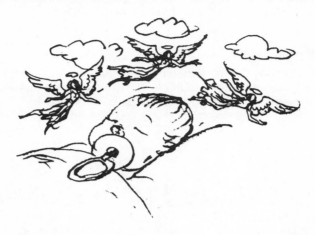

Attention-seeking

It could be that he wants attention. I was always astonished at the number of perfectly sane and apparently kindly people who would encourage me not to go to my screaming baby on the grounds that 'he just wants attention'. It seemed perfectly reasonable to me that if he wanted attention he should have it; after all, I've wanted attention often enough myself and feel very down-in-the-dumps if no one comes up with the goods. Attention is important for a baby. No one would say: 'For heaven's sake leave the baby to cry; he's just freezing cold/starving/dying of a fever/in agony.' So if your baby cries because he wants attention, then give it to him.

Swaddling

Although binding a baby firmly is not common in this country, some babies are soothed by being wrapped up tightly in a shawl (not *too* tightly, of course) so that their arms can't move much. It's worth trying this, at least temporarily.

Soothing noises and rocking

Babies are lulled by the most peculiar sounds, from the buzzing of an electric clock to the whir of a vacuum cleaner. Some parents find that jamming their babies in the back of the car and driving them a few times round the block to get them to calm down and go to sleep often works. If you're a cyclist, however, the old lullaby method could work, particularly if you rock him very gently at the same time. Don't swing him too hard – the best rock is a swing of 2¾″ at one-second intervals. A radio put on very quietly by the door can reassure some babies, too.

Overtiredness

It's important to distinguish an over-tired cry from an angry cry if you can. Many mothers instantly say: 'Oh, he's tired' the minute a baby starts to bawl and then spend a frustrating half-hour trying to get a furiously active, alert and eager baby to sleep, with no success. You can usually tell when a baby is over-tired, however, by his red face, heavy eye-lids and the particularly reckless kind of crying, which will be ended in a deep sleep after quarter of an hour.

Boredom

It's all very well for you, with your brand-new baby books to read and a phone by your side, but he, poor chap, has only the dismal white walls of his carrycot to stimulate him. No wonder he cries. Company and action is what the bored baby is after and there's nothing he'll like better than dragging you out to large stores during the sales, his eyes popping out of his head as you stumble up escalators, carrycot on your head, wheels in one hand and him in the other. A trip to the park, the sandpit, the shops or even tea with another mother and baby can work wonders in getting him healthily tired by the evening. You, certainly, will be completely whacked.

Wind and colic

No one really knows if wind in a baby really does upset him. Is he comforted by the soothing effect of being patted and stroked or is that burp a real relief from gastric agony? Gripe water soothes some babies. But the answer to a windy or colicky child is really rather like religion. It doesn't matter what you believe as long as you believe in something. When a child has colic, particularly in the evenings, there is really not much you can do except your best. If you're desperate, leave him for quarter of an hour, as Dr Spock suggests, have a drink and try to relax before trying again. Of course, you may not have to.

One of the best ways of dealing with crying is to listen to it analytically before rushing to comfort the baby. You may get to know your baby's cries and learn to differentiate between furious crying, miserable crying, crying with pain or fright or tiredness. Or could he be just 'trying it on'. I don't believe that a baby can be so cunning that he can actually 'try it on', but there's a school of thought that believes that babies are just little monsters waiting to catch you out. The little chap may be only a week old and screaming with hunger, but there's always some knowing busy-body who will peer into the cot unsympathetically and say: 'Ha! You crafty little devil!' They regard their babies – and, later, their children – as villainous opponents; their job is always to have 'eyes at the back of the head' in case the baby catches them out, and they hold that a good mother is the one who can outwit her crafty baby most of the time.

Those who are more sensitive (like you) will find this approach unhelpful to say the least, and you'll get more satisfaction by trying to tune into the baby and really think about what it is he is crying for. However, it's always easy to tell mothers to learn their babies' different cries. I could never tell one cry from another: all my baby's cries sounded the same to me – angry and utterly miserable – and they always made me feel absolutely awful.

However, even the least sensitive among us should be able to recognise her own baby's cry as distinct from another's – but be prepared for that awful moment when, out to dinner with another mother, there is a cry from upstairs at which both of you rise to your feet with a smug, maternal smile and an: 'Ah, that's little Sasha/Johnnie – I can *always* tell . . .' and it turns out to be the cat.

A few weeks will at least give you enough experience to prevent quite a bit of crying. You will just *know* that he will be reduced to tears when an aged friend of the family arrives, and, best hat bobbing and face curled up into a grotesque grin, sticks her hand out and says: 'Will he come to me, then? Will he? Will you come to me? Will he? Come, come to your auntie . . . !'

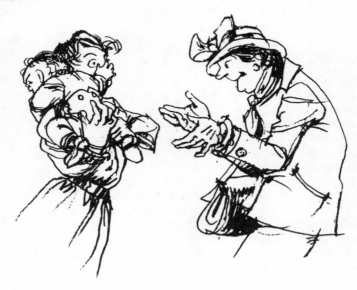

You may know that he'll cry if you ever leave the room and so rather than let things get to that point, you must hoist him up and take him with you – to answer the bell, feed the cat or even to go to the loo.

You also know he'll cry at points when you can't do anything about it. A friend who comes round and gossips on and on can make your blood pressure rise as the time goes by and you *know* that the baby will cry unless you give him some reassuring attention. (Indeed, it's quite uncanny how the baby will often cry at the moment when, were you not a civilised, controlled adult, you would spontaneously cry yourself.) You may be fairly sure that he'll cry at the worst moments, too – like when the pediatrician wants to examine him, when your best friend presents him with a beautiful Victorian coral and silver teething rattle, when you're longing to get him to sleep early so as not to miss the movie round the corner, and on a long and boring car journey, just as you approach the rush-hour traffic jam.

A little later he will cry because he daren't go to other people – the clinging cry. Take him to a sandpit and the minute you dump him in the sand, he starts to yell. The answer to this is not to force it, with mutterings of: 'Be independent and enjoy yourself, for God's sake!' under your breath, but to resign yourself to it. The moment you tell yourself that you are doomed, like a weary St Christopher, to carry him for ever, is the moment he will start wriggling to get off your knee and crawl away on his own.

The crying baby can wreck friendships. Outsiders always see – or think they see – so clearly how your baby should be handled, and how foolishly you're handling yours, that they finally start telling you what to do. 'Pick him up, can't you; can't you see, he's longing to be picked up?' says some exasperated other mum. Or, 'Smack, go on, show him who's boss, he's got to learn, he's *asking* for it.' Or, 'Go on, give him a lolly, he wants it so much.' It's not only important to try to remain as unaffected by this as possible, but also to choke back any similar criticisms you may have of the other mother's methods of handling *her* crying baby, unless she is being extremely and obviously cruel.

You can always see how seriously a mother takes crying by whether she has a Baby Alarm or not. This is a sort of extension of the umbilical cord, a microphone attached to the baby's cot, the noise from the cot being transmitted by a wire and battery to a loudspeaker near the parents. Owners of this machine are usually parents who are worried about crying and often have the machine turned up so loud that every meal is spent to the accompaniment of heavy breathing through the loud-speaker. Each time the baby turns it sounds as if his room has been upturned by an earthquake; every time he coughs it sounds as if he's being strangled by a maniac in the dark.

Remember that it is not only crying that is transmitted on this machine. Sudden loud voices picked up from radio taxis or police cars shouting: 'Roger, over and out!' may send the parents into fits of panic thinking their child has been attacked by burglars (or perhaps has suddenly started from his cot in a fit of confidence to practise a newly acquired vocabulary).

Having used a baby alarm myself and driven the whole family to distraction with it (it would be better titled a Parent Alarm, come to think of it), I can't recommend it unless you live in a castle or a four-storey Victorian house where you really can't hear the baby in its room from where you sit in the evenings.

In all, the best thing to do with a crying baby is to think twice before running to it – and then run to it as quickly as possible. And remember that a baby who never cried would be a frightening and worrying thing.

9
Feeding

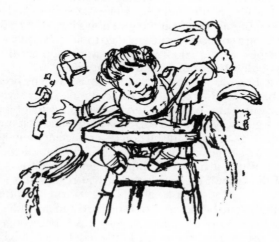

Considering that in some cultures babies live healthily on milk alone for a year at least, it's ridiculous that Western mothers spend so much time panicking about feeding.

Generations of rickety children have bred this obsession with vitamin drops, solid food, real fruit juice and a horror of those worst of all unhealthy vices, 'biscuits and sweets'. What you give your child and how much he takes *is* important, of course, but very few mothers have got feeding into perspective.

It all starts when someone sidles up on the first day after your baby has been born and mutters: 'Breast or bottle?' There's one group of women who could be called the Breast Brigade. They tend to be extremists. They badger you to breast-feed the baby, claiming that milk like mother makes is better for the baby, psychologically necessary and that, above all, it is Nature's Way. (But, as we all know, Nature's Way is not always the best way.) The Breast Brigade have a battery of 'breast accessories' – the idea of which, out of context, may make you want to throw up, though you may actually need them when it comes to it. These ladies are all for nipple massage, false teats to aid problem feeding, nipple shields, milk ducts, nipple cream and feeding bras. Whenever you say you breast-feed your baby, they all stick out their bosoms and look proud and happy, pat you on the shoulder and say: 'Good girl!' The longer you can feed your baby, the more pleased they are. 'You fed him for eighteen months?' they would say to me, a manic breast-feeder at the time. 'Wonderful! Splendid!'

The other group, the Bottle Brigade, argue that bottles are more convenient. There are none of those agonising problems of wondering if you have enough milk for the baby, because if the bottle runs out you can simply make some more. You can *see* how much milk the baby has drunk, too, if you're using a bottle, and that can be reassuring. And anyone can give him a bottle, while only you can give him a breast. If he wakes up in the night wanting a comforting suck he'll go to sleep happily with a bottle chucked into the cot from a doorway. If you want to go out, the babysitter can give the bottle while you dance the night away.

The Breast Brigade argue that, as far as is known, breast milk is fractionally better for the baby than artificial milk. They say that breast-feeding gets your figure back quicker. They also say that breast-feeding mothers can't get away from the baby too long – and that this is a good thing (but no one can prove this. If you're a reluctant mum anyway, and there are lots of quite good mothers who aren't wild about the baby stage of childhood, it might be a bad thing to get yourself too tied to the demands of the baby if the result is that you resent him.) The Breast Brigade also say that breasts are lovely, warm, comfortable and comforting things and bottles are cold and hard and horrible. This is true – but one of the reasons we might believe this is because *we* associate breasts with happy feeding times; bottle-fed babies might associate *bottles* with feeding time and see them as beautiful, clear and fresh and swoon at the appetising smell of a rubber teat.

For some mothers, due to circumstances or emotional taboos, there's simply no choice in the matter of breast *v.* bottle-feeding, so the decision is made for them – and no one should feel guilty or inadequate because they aren't able to breast-feed. A lot of modern propaganda suggests that breast-feeding is the first maternal duty, which is plainly ridiculous. And the reason *I* preferred breast-feeding was simply because it was more convenient. You don't have to sterilise any equipment or go in for those heating gadgets; and at night you can just haul the baby into bed, lie on your side and doze while he feeds. I'll never forget the sight of some of my friends, head-to-toe in rubber gloves, plastic aprons, plunging into kitchens full of steam and counting out spoonfuls of dried milk loudly so they wouldn't make a mistake, and then heating up needles to enlarge the holes in the teats. (Some of these mums were still sterilising long after the baby had started a diet of fresh fluff, dead leaves, sand and grubby crusts picked up off the street.)

But in the very short-term, bottle-feeding is easier. It takes most first mothers at least a week (and sometimes quite an upsetting week at that) just to get the hang of breast-feeding. Breast-feeding isn't just a matter of

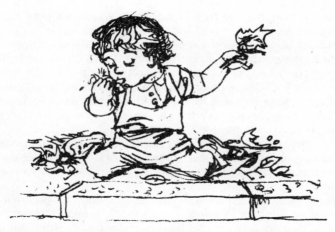

'A diet of fresh fluff, dead leaves, sand and grubby crusts picked up off the street'

jamming the baby up to the breast and getting out a thriller to read over the top of his head. In the early days, just after he's born, the milk comes into the breasts and, depending on your physical make-up, you'll either have a few drops and give up or turn into a huge milking-machine, breasts swelling up to a size that would qualify you instantly for a job in a strip joint. No bra will fit, you wake up surrounded by pools of milk, smelling like a dairy, and as you walk you leave behind you a trail of drips. Whenever the baby cries, your nipples respond by starting up like pistols spurting milk instead of bullets.

If your breasts get too uncomfortably large, you're recommended to 'express' your milk, a term that makes you feel more like a dairy than ever. The hospital will probably produce an electric milking machine which drags the nipple in and out, squeezing the milk out drop by drop (and which, as you might imagine, can be extremely uncomfortable). The best relief is to massage the sides of your breasts with flannels soaked in hot water, and, lying in the bath, expressing the milk by hand under the water. Don't express too much milk, though; the more you express, the more is produced and you can end up the morning after even more uncomfortable than when you started.

There are often problems, too, with your nipples. Sore nipples are common as are, sometimes, small or inverted nipples. The answer to the vanishing nipple is a large, plastic, cup-shaped object called a nipple shield, shaped to make your tiny nipples push out enough for the baby to be able to get a hold. The only embarrassment is when a visiting relation or, worse still, an old boyfriend, giving you a big congratulatory hug, is alarmed to hear the strange clunk of plastic breast against the button of his overcoat.

If you're having problems in hospital, seek out a kindly nurse (you can't be so unlucky as to have none) and badger her until you have mastered the art.

Even at home, you may *still* experience problems. If you're fussed, give yourself a strong drink, turn on the telly and turn off all the lights and boot everyone out so that you can relax properly with the baby. Panic will only produce less milk, not more; this is why a bottle at the ready is always helpful in the first stages of breast-feeding, as you don't feel so totally responsible for satisfying your baby's hunger . . . and, as a result, you're more likely to give a better feed.

It might be thought that once the breast or bottle fuss had been sorted out, you deserve a break. Not so. Only too soon will that same person who murmured: 'Breast or bottle,' slink up again to ask: 'Are you demand feeding?'

I always hated the expression 'demand feeding'. I'd prefer it to be called 'ask-feeding' or 'feeding on request'. Demand-feeding has a pejorative ring to it, as if the baby were a badly brought-up, bad-mannered and intrinsically nasty little tyrant. It all goes with that idea that babies are born with the devil inside them – and that they are guilty until proved innocent. Most unjust.

The opposite to demand feeding is routine feeding, which sounds easier but often means the baby crying for ages in the most irritating and upsetting way. There's obviously some way between being a slave to your baby or it being a slave to you and this is what you should aim for. Try to organise some kind of loose regime (feeding every two to three hours in the first few weeks if he's a hungry baby) and let him have a feed with half an hour either way of your schedule.

But as you begin to organise some kind of time-table and think you're home and dry at last, the trouble-maker appears again, when the baby is about eight months old, simply to say, casually: 'Oh, isn't he on to solids yet?'

'Solids' is an exaggeration for the strained mush that passes for food in the world of babies. Go round any supermarket and you will see hundreds of jars and tins all of which look deliciously tempting, with bonny babies with quiffs like toupees on the tops of their heads grinning from the labels. Some have enticing titles: 'Peach and Grape Delight', 'Egg, Bacon, Sausage, Tomato and Kipper Breakfast'. But when you open them they all taste almost exactly the same, are greyish in colour and, to a tin, disgusting (at least *I* think so). This does not mean that the baby won't eat them. After all, this is a baby who is going to grow into a little boy or girl whose favourite dish is sausages covered with marmalade rounded off by a chocolate spread and peanut butter sandwich topped by HP sauce. No wonder he's keen on this tinned sludge, punctuated by the odd green speck that passes for a pea and the stray piece of orange-coloured string that is, hopefully, a carrot.

If you've given birth to a human dustbin you're free of further problems – a baby who jumps up and down with excitement in his high

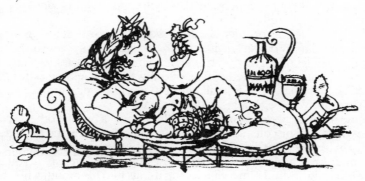

'Peach and Grape Delight'

chair at the sight of a couple of tins, not to mention yesterday's left-overs of cold Brussels sprouts, and crams biscuits and rusks into his face until you can scarcely see his eyes. Most food is thrown on the floor as a matter of course, as well. Like a king who has to have a taster before he touches his food, most babies won't look at their sausages until they've tested them well for floorability; only then will they be considered fit for baby consumption.

But if your baby is a gourmet who sneers at 'Nut, Honey and Lemon Pudding' and demands to see the manager when it's presented on his plate, a baby who, when offered a spoonful of mashed banana, firmly closes his mouth and looks interestedly to the left and right – then you've got trouble.

A baby who doesn't eat turns all of us into Jewish mommas. 'Eat, eat, my boy,' you hear yourself saying. 'You will never grow big and strong like your papa. I make you special dumplings and you don't eat them? You're not well? Eat, eat . . .' A baby who won't eat forces us out to buy baby Mouli-graters, finds us grinding up concoctions of bananas, carrots or yesterday's supper and hoping he'll eat that. Maybe he will; maybe he won't. Most likely he'll stuff himself with yesterday's pureed coq-au-vin one day, but next day, if you make it for him specially (and there's *nothing* a worried mother won't do) he'll suddenly go all yawny and push it away.

Go to the clinic and you will get no reassurance. 'What about finger foods?' they will suggest, brightly, thrusting a diet sheet into your hands which gives a list of tempting appetisers like strips of marmite-covered bread, enticing slivers of cucumber and carrot, toast cunningly soaked in egg, crackers covered with peanut butter (so nourishing). They will declare that you have what is politely known as an Independent Baby, or one that prefers to eat with his hands. Give him bread and butter and he'll pick the butter off with his fingers; make the mistake of offering him peas and he will eat by picking them up in his tiny fingers one by wretched one. Most likely your Independent Baby will simply use his hands to push away anything offered.

The answer to this problem is: don't worry. Unless he's losing weight drastically it simply doesn't matter if he doesn't eat. He's not ill; he just has a small appetite. And if he doesn't eat the right things, that doesn't matter very much either, provided you're offering him something other than sweet biscuits. Many children all over the world never eat meat; Henry VIII very rarely ate vegetables. It doesn't matter.

Some babies survive on one small sausage a week; others cram themselves with biscuits, steaks and ice-creams, grabbing the odd bag of apples in between. It takes a lot to make a baby die, certainly if he always has some food available. What *will* upset him, however, is if you are always fussing around him trying to pop things into his mouth when he's yawning.

The irony of feeding is that at the end of the first year you go back to the beginning again. The very art it took so long to master in the first place now has to be unlearnt. 'Weaning' is the word, and while the books may say that to wean a baby from the breast 'you just cut out the midday breast feed for a fortnight, and substitute a cup or bottle, then the evening one and so on,' some babies get hooked on tits and have withdrawal symptoms, screaming and yelling and being thoroughly miserable. One of the reasons in favour of getting a baby used to a bottle from the beginning is that it makes weaning much easier. And try to wean quite *early*, at about six months, however much pleasure you're getting from feeding, because it does get more difficult as the baby gets older. Difficulties in weaning are rarely mentioned, but nearly all doctors have a few late weaners on their books, and their mothers begin to get worried when the baby is around eighteen months. In some countries children sometimes feed until the age of four and their parents are obliged to put bitter aloes on their nipples to kick them of the habit.

There is no need to go this far. But remember that usually it's not just the baby who gets hooked on feeding. Your problems start when *you* get hooked on it as well, and, deep down, you don't want to stop. Never wean when you're feeling low or depressed; and once you find yourself in a confident mood, drop a feed a day for a fortnight at least. It's sometimes easiest to wean when you're on holiday and can spend a lot of time jollying the baby out of any distress. When you're busy it's always so much easier to give in to a feed than to work at persuading him to accept a cup or bottle instead.

From the moment weaning begins, the whole feeding process goes into reverse. Next you have to cut out the tins, then the rusks and get him eating ordinary meals. Just reassure yourself that by the time he's thirty and starting to worry about long-term health, he'll be giving up all the eggs you so carefully encouraged him to eat during the first year. But at least he'll have to do it by himself.

10

Travelling and Visiting

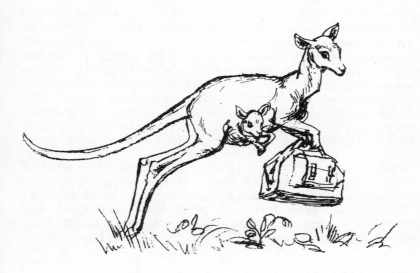

You probably remember the days when, arriving at the station of your destination, you excused your haggard looks and fraught expression saying: 'My God, what a journey ... there was this frightful *baby* in my compartment, you see ...'

Now this 'frightful baby' is yours. *You* are the woman roaming down the corridors of trains while passengers look up in horror and draw down the blinds of their compartments when they see the Small Bundle in your arms. It is to keep *you* away that they litter the carriage with luggage to make it look occupied, while they slump lengthways across the seat, pretending to sleep, to disguise the existence of vacant seats. It is *you* who hear their sighs of relief as you pass, while they pick up their papers again and thank their lucky stars their journey is now safe.

Travelling with a baby is such a labour that you may well be tempted to stay in during the first year. The baby is small but taking him from A to B is like the circus coming to town. He needs a carrycot; a large bag of accessories – extra nappies, extra cardigan, fresh clothes, bottle, dummy, toy, plastic bag for dirty nappy, cotton wool, tissues or wipes and probably foldable carrycot wheels. And as he gets older he gets heavier and you find you have more in common with St Christopher than you ever suspected.

However, go into the outside world you *must*, simply to keep yourself sane.

First steps

In the early weeks the sling is best. It feels much more comfortable to carry him close to you, as you have been for the last nine months, after all. It's surely much nicer for him to be close to you, too, and you'll benefit from a feeling of independence that you won't get with a pram. You will also be relieved of baby-snatching fears as he is with you all the time (the irrational fear is always with you even though it's one of the very rarest occurrences), and he will prefer to accompany you round the supermarket to stare at the colours rather than being left outside to gaze at the sky. Be sure to try out the slings with a friend before making your first trip, however. They are very simple to rig up *after* you have got the hang of them.

When he's older, use the back-pack, which also has the advantage of being a hit with those husbands who revel in the tough, rough, hiking appearance it gives them compared to the Flora margarine-ish image of a bloke wheeling a pram. Back-packs are also good on rough country ground where a pram would be too bumpy, and they're useful, too, to stuff your sweaters and sandwiches in if you go for a long hike.

Prams and pushchairs

Pram pushing, like basket-weaving, is a skill. Some mothers get it taped after the first week but it's no easy task to master. Pushing the machine into shops always needs help from other people – usually little old ladies, the sort for whom you used to be holding the door open yourself. And the handle of the pram is always far too low, so that if you are more than one inch taller than Princess Margaret you have to learn the Groucho Marx Pram Walk.

To get into shops on your own, the trick is to back into the shop by pushing the door open with your bottom, or to go forward by pushing the pram against the door of the shop; then, with your right hand, giving it a shove and racing in quickly before it crashes back, either onto the baby's head or your right elbow. Initially it involves a lot of bruising; it is good practice for a trainee stuntman though I suspect most old hands would beg to be taken back to drive motorcycles through hoops of fire.

Which pram to get depends on how much you care about what other people think and how well off you are. Most mums bear in mind that they won't be using the pram for longer than a year and, by scouring the ads in

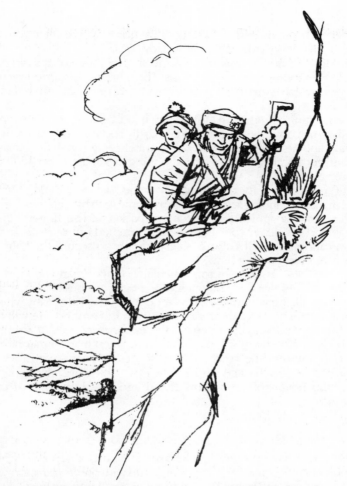

'A hit with those husbands who revel in the tough, rough, hiking appearance'

tobacconists' windows, searching the noticeboards in nursery schools and clinics or badgering friends, pick up something second-hand. But if you're out to buy something new, there's a huge choice.

Nannies in Kensington Gardens sport baby carriages like broughams with double-hoods that seem permanently to be shivering slightly, so well-sprung are they. Inside lies a tiny baby practically lost among the linen sheets and Shetland pram blankets. Do *not* get one of these unless you have extra space in the garage, a huge hall or a disused ballroom to park it in.

At the bottom of the social perambulating scale is the basic carrycot on wheels, the second-hand bike of perambulating. This is a fairly bumpy number and even on surfaces as smooth as gravel will result in your baby having a fairly jerky ride. He usually enjoys this.

The Minis of the pram world are the snappy little collapsible prams suitable for nipping around the shops. These are sophisticated carrycots on wheels which convert into pushchairs later. The drawback is that they weigh a ton.

When getting a pram, don't forget you need a space for your shopping as well as the baby. Sometimes there's hardly room for the baby during a big shop and he'll peer out rather desperately between the bananas and the joint; get a pram that has a wire shopping rack that can be slung at the bottom.

Later, get a basket for the pushchair at the back so you don't have to perform mad balancing acts on your way home with baskets weighing the handles down so much that one more packet of fish fingers tips the balance and results in your baby being launched out of his seat like a human cannon ball. (It's always safer, actually, to secure the baby with straps, wherever you put him.)

The transition from pram to pushchair is bigger than you think, and there's no doubt that baby buggies, being light, are best. But now, from being safely facing you in a pram at about waist level, the baby will have his back to you and sits about one foot from the ground. He will try to poke hungry Alsatian guard dogs in the eye and acquire, in a shop, six Mars bars, one bottle of whisky and a purse lifted from someone else's basket, by the time he reaches the cash desk. Be on guard for other people's shopping baskets and brief-cases, which are always held at exactly the height of your baby's head and are therefore extremely dangerous.

Public transport

While you may have mastered walking about with a baby, going by public transport is a different story. Everything to do with public transport works against a mother and baby. The left-luggage space on new buses (where you're obliged to leave the pushchair) is in the centre of the vehicle, making every trip awkward and irritating; underground stations are a maze of long flights of unscaleable stairs, escalators and automatic ticket-machines. You'll also notice that the gap that appears between the platform and the waiting train is exactly the right size for a baby to slip through onto the electric rails below.

This is no time for false pride or declarations of women's lib. Since the underground, particularly during the day, is usually peopled by men, you must seek help from jolly fatherly blokes who, if you're lucky, will just pick up the entire pushchair plus the astonished baby in one hand and zip up to the top of the stairs while asking how old the little chap is before you have puffed half way up. These are Other Dads, and transport is the only area in which they will feature in your life at all.

Car

If you're lucky enough to go by car *do take care*. Install carrycot straps to fix the cot to the back seat firmly, and strap the baby in so that he doesn't spring out and hurt himself if you stop suddenly. Keep some toys in the carrycot or preferably a cradle gym just for the car to keep him occupied during traffic jams. It is an impossible and upsetting business to concentrate on driving and calm the baby down in the back at the same time.

Never let the baby travel with other small children under two and a half at the back for fear that they might start bopping him just as you get on to the M1. And remember it's now against the law to travel with your baby in the front seat of the car. The driver only has to brake suddenly for your baby's head to be smashed onto the dashboard.

Later he will outgrow the carrycot. You will know that moment has arrived either when you need a giant shoe-horn to squeeze his toes into it and his head is jammed into his stomach like a passenger trying to take a nap in an aeroplane seat, or you'll be alarmed when, travelling down the middle lane of the motorway, you glance into your suddenly shaded mirror to see what dark lorry is over-taking you only to find the laughing face of your baby who is actually standing up in the back and reaching for the gears. This is the moment to acquire a baby car seat, usually a little fake leather affair that attaches at the back, shaped like a piece of furniture out of one of James Bond's penthouse flats, all trendy and Swedish-looking. Put the baby in it and he looks surprisingly like a small executive for a sharp property firm.

When he outgrows this, or if you let him loose in the back, do get a child-proof locking device on the doors. However, it is much better to install proper seatbelts for children in the back.

Never put the carrycot or young child in the hatch of a hatch-back car. This area is known in the trade as the 'crumple-zone' and is designed to squash itself up into the back of the back seat when hit by the bad driver behind you.

Train

If you take a train, start early. It takes ages to realise that babies add hours to travelling. When you pack you'll find it very easy to forget to take anything for yourself, so busy are you packing for the baby; this is the moment to make a list of 'yours' and 'his', and do remember that almost all his extras – like disposable nappies – can be bought wherever you're going; but your one un-stained dress is irreplaceable, so don't forget it. You have to start for trains at the same time as your parents used to, fussily early, to take account of nappy changes, temper tantrums, requests for drinks and lugging wheels and bags of nappies down platforms. If you are extra early you can find a completely empty compartment – much the best because no one in their right minds will join you and your offspring.

Aeroplanes

Most aeroplanes have excellent baby services, unlike any other forms of transport, and, on long trips, will provide a bassinet that suspends from the ceiling, if you warn them in advance. Sucking a dummy or a lolly during take-off will relieve the baby of pain in his ears, and he will probably be barely aware that you have left the ground.

It might just be worth taking extra care, however, before you take the baby on the aeroplane at all. It is fine if you're off to a sophisticated country with excellent hospitals and medical care, but I personally would be very dubious of taking a *very* small baby even to somewhere as nearby as a charming village in Tuscany without good travel insurance. Babies can get very ill very quickly and most English mums find a lot of medical care abroad not up to British standards. Ask your travel agent about insurance schemes that ensure an immediate flight back in emergencies.

Outings

With a baby, however, it is often better to travel, even hopelessly, than to arrive. Remember that babies are extremely sensitive to different atmospheres and if he's good as gold at home, he may play up on holiday or in a stranger's house (and vice-versa). The embarrassed phrase 'He isn't always like this' is one a mum can expect to repeat again and again throughout her travels, whether he's crying fit to burst or suddenly killing himself laughing when he's never smiled before in his life.

So wherever you go, do take quite a lot of familiar gear with you, even his own food. It's always upsetting and embarrassing to find yourself with a hostess who's taken immense trouble to re-arrange the house to suit the baby, with piles of bricks, borrowed high-chairs, specially mashed-up lunch, specially made-up cot – and then to see the baby reject everything in turn. He won't eat, he won't sleep, he won't play and it's quite clear to everyone, including your hostess, that he just wants to go right home, at once.

I might add that this doesn't always happen, babies being unpredictable creatures. Often your baby will suddenly 'take' to another person and her habits, her squashed bananas, her toys, her cot and her house, and behave far better than he ever does at home, to the point of going to sleep without fuss after lunch and eating all his tea. I always remember insisting that my baby would never dream of sitting in a strange high-chair and that he absolutely *had* to sit on my knee, until the furious hostess snatched him out of my arms, placed him in the high-chair and what did the little wretch do? Cry? Not a bit of it. He slid into it happily as if he were saying: 'Why haven't we got one of these *splendidly* comfortable contraptions at home . . . *so* convenient and handy, *so* easy to keep clean' (passing a finger delightedly over the Formica tray) 'so elegantly designed. Ah – and an amusing plastic bib, too, how I *wish* my mother kept one of these . . .' He ate three courses of a meal that he would have spurned at home, fell into a deep, contented slumber – and my wails of, 'But he's not usually like this,' didn't convince my hostess, who looked at me accusingly, suspecting (oh, so wrongly) that I'd never offered him interesting meals or high-chairs or bibs in his life.

Social occasions

When the baby is very small, you will probably take him with you when you and your partner go out in the evenings. To be honest, this is not a very satisfactory procedure. Nearly everyone does it, because babysitters are expensive and he is, in the first-year, quite light enough to carry easily. But unless you move in very liberal circles, among friends who genuinely enjoy kids being around in the evenings, a baby is about as welcome to the dinner party as a playful dog. Your hostess will peer into the carrycot with rude haste, see his eyes are shut and declare: 'Great! He's asleep! You can stick him in the spare room! It's right up five flights so he won't be disturbed.'

The phrase 'he won't be disturbed' really means 'We won't be disturbed'. Very few babies are disturbed by noise; if they're tired they sleep and if they're miserable, bored or unhappy, they cry. But all hosts and hostesses are disturbed by the cries of a baby at their dinner party which is why, from 3 p.m. on, they have put on the electric fire to warm up the baby's sleeping quarters, usually a room which is always so far away from the dining-room that not even the most sensitively attuned mother would hear him.

When the baby is older and starts crawling or walking, he becomes positively anti-social. However quiet and self-contained and charming your child is – and to *you* he's almost certain to be the most fascinating and entertaining person around – children are taboo round the supper table in England because of the general terror that the baby might detract from the star guest or burp just before the punchline of a funny story.

However you feel about this (I much prefer the French way of allowing children and babies up with the grown-ups), you must resign yourself to the fact that you won't be able to change people's views here; babies aren't popular in the evenings and it is socially far more acceptable to arrive very late with a sleeping baby than punctually with an active one.

Babysitters

Schoolchildren are usually eager to baby-sit and are reasonably cheap, while agencies are much more expensive, but more reliable. The law about leaving children is difficult, incidentally. If anything ghastly happens to children under sixteen on their own you can be had up for criminal neglect. So see your babysitters are all over sixteen. If you're desperate, try driving your baby to a friend's house to sleep there, and pick him up on your way back when he is asleep. Baby-sitting circles with other couples are a cheap way of getting your babysitting done (but you have to baby-sit back for them, of course). Never take a baby-sitter without references. Leave your phone number and the phone number of your doctor in case of emergency, and, to be on the safe side, give your baby-sitter a ring when you arrive at your destination. You can then check the number you have given her, check that she is still at your home, and check the baby is all right.

Travelling is an effort, but it is a pity *not* to go and visit grandparents at Christmas or to go to the seaside in the summer just because of the daunting effort of taking the baby. Once you've done it once or twice, it will become, like having babies, easier.

Travelling is only the lesser of two evils, the other being to stay permanently at home. If a baby could talk he might want to go out much less every day, the simple visits to the shops in the morning and park in the afternoons being ample stimulation. It's only *you* who needs to make at least one wild expedition a week, to friends, to a hairdresser, to a sale, in order to keep yourself that calm, friendly and stimulating companion that your baby needs when you are both at home. Well, calmish.

11

The Working Mother

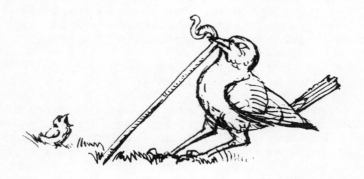

If you feel you have to work for money then weigh up the advantages of full-time employment with social security or supplementary benefit. Once you've paid for fares, lunch and someone to look after the child you will probably only just break even. But if you're lucky enough to have a working partner, then unless you are at starvation point or the first woman MP in a mining constitutency I really can't see the point of going right back to a nine-to-five job when your baby is six months old. I mean, why on earth did you have the baby in the first place? However, for a lot of mothers, part-time work, from the moment you start to feel bored and trapped, is essential.

Not going or going back to work is one of the crucial decisions in the modern woman's life because more women these days are better and further educated to work at jobs which are careers as well. And then, suddenly, we have children and have to give it all up. Some do, willingly and happily, but others feel that the door has closed on the great world and we are right back in women's traditional role. What was the point of all that education and work? Usually any kind of going back to work will be a compromise – more to make ends meet or to satisfy an inner need than an ascension of the job's ladder.

It's true that other mothers at this point may fill you with guilt by saying: 'Well, I can't see the point of working when they're young. The years before five are crucial, anyway. They're only young once, after all – it's not fair on them.' But you must reply that the theory that the first five years are crucial is under attack and that you are only 'twenty', 'thirty' or 'forty' once and it's not fair on you either.

It is possible that one of the reasons you long for a change of scene is that you are one of those mothers who find tiny babies maddening. (Some mums, on the other hand, just adore babies and find their seven- and eight-year-olds a pain in the neck, while others really only feel they've got the hang of motherhood when their children are teenagers.)

If you're not one of nature's baby-lovers then it probably is more than fair on your baby for you to get a part-time job. You will be better tempered when you get back from work, you won't be tempted to blame your baby for your feelings of isolation and loneliness; and it's better for a baby to be left *part* of the day with an affectionate minder than all day with a bad-tempered, resentful mother.

Before you take a job, though, be sure you know exactly *why* you're doing it. Do you really need the money, for instance (if you're taking a full-time job)? – because the baby won't notice if his clothes are brand new or second-hand or whether he has a well-sprung pram or a battered old carrycot on wheels. It's only worth working for money if you either need it desperately or think that you wouldn't be able to stand life without a bit of comfort for yourself.

Or are you just going to work because you feel so stricken with guilt when you hear about all those expert mums who bring up four kids with one hand, sit on charity committees in their spare time and make their own jam, run boutiques and take courses at the Open University with the other? These mums are rare birds; they always have help in the shape of an au pair or housekeeper and, to be honest, I always wonder whether they *do* bring up their children very well.

Or are you going to work because you feel you're no longer the bright, amusing, well-informed girl you were a few years back? There's a lot of talk, when you have a baby, about how you're going to turn into a vegetable, and this can happen. But an obsessive interest in the qualities of different dried milks or what the grocer's grandchild weighed at birth should not necessarily be the sign of a vegetable or a bore. There are nappy bores – and there are racing-car bores, and make-your-own-wine bores and political bores. But there is nothing in the subject of babies that's necessarily dull and no one should apologise for telling a story about a baby; they should only apologise if they tell a boring story about a baby.

Or are you going to work because, although you love your baby, you don't want to look after him *all* the time? It is a seven-day-a-week job of at least twelve hours a day, even with a perfect baby, and no one should be blamed for wanting to take a few hours off now and again.

If you can't find a part-time job, don't sniff at Saturday jobs. You might even make some money as your partner can look after the baby, which will mean they get to know each other better. Because whatever you do, your biggest problem is: who will look after the baby?

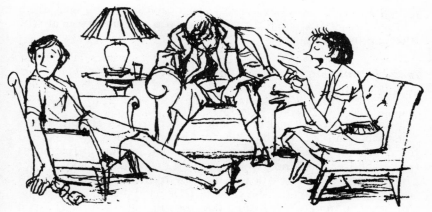

'There are nappy bores . . .'

The babyminder

This is a word that conjures up a dark, dank room packed with crowds of small children lit by the flickering light of a huge old black and white television set. Some *are* like that, so be scrupulous about finding the right minder for your baby.

First ring your local council or put an advertisement in a tobacconist's window or your local paper. Although it is important to find out whether the baby-minder is registered, don't be afraid to back your own personal hunches. Visit her in her home, see how many toys she has, subtract several points for a giant colour telly dominating the room, ask what she gives the children to eat, examine her bathroom, get two references from her and ask for the phone number of a mother of at least one of the other children she looks after. Finally, send the baby's dad round without giving her notice. He can claim he was 'just dropping by' – and will spot whether she was putting on a good front when you saw her or whether she's always charming, clean and friendly.

If you feel that although her flat is spotless, her children are happy and the place is covered with educational toys, *but* there's something funny about her eyes/smile/expression that you can't quite put your finger on, *don't* send your baby to her. It's worth taking a lot of trouble finding the right person, and, hopefully, your baby will be able to go to her for different periods during the day right up to when he is three years old and going to nursery school (for which, by the way, you should be putting his name down right now as they get very booked up).

Day nursery

Usually you can only get a place if you are a single parent, or the child is deprived in some way. Day nurseries take babies all day usually, from 7.30 a.m. to 6.30 p.m., and you can find out if you have any in your area by ringing your local council.

Amiable teenager

These are willing but not very reliable characters. If you live in town you will find that once you have a baby you will meet a lot of them, anxious to take the baby out for a walk or do little motherly chores. The problem is that, though full of amiability, they are low on initiative. If you have to resort to one of these, meet her own mother, get lots of references (preferably from her school), make sure she's over sixteen, and give her a rigid plan of what she is to do with the baby from the moment she leaves your house until the time she gets back. Demand that she goes to the park, gives him tea at a certain time, does the shopping – anything to keep her busy all the time she is out. Give her a list of don'ts (like don't take the baby in a car, have friends round to your house, etc.) and check up from time to time by ringing up to see that everything is going as planned.

Amiable teenagers should really only be used as second strings when all else has gone wrong; I would never like to depend on one myself; I remember too well how responsible I seemed as a teenager. And how irresponsible I really was.

Unmarried mother

It is tempting to let the only spare room in your house to an unmarried mother who will not only do all the housework and know the ropes as far as babies go, but also provide your offspring with 'a little friend'. Remember, though, that unmarried mothers, like all mothers, are rightly only really concerned with the well-being of their own baby, and as it gets older, yours will get pushed more and more into the shade. Before you commit yourself to any arrangement like this, consult a solicitor and the Rent Act. If you suddenly turned against her, it might be *very* difficult to get rid of her quickly.

Mother's help

Mothers' helps are living-in girls who've just left school. There is a lot to be said for these because they speak the language and they are not expensive; but they are young and may well get home-sick.

Au Pair

If you can afford it and get a good one you are very lucky. But au pairs usually can't be vetted before they arrive, unless you go to an agency which specialises in dissatisfied au pairs who wish to move on from their family during their year in England. Yours will speak little English. She won't stay longer than a year and you may be lucky if she stays a year at all. She has to be fed and paid; she has to be spoken to and listened to, to improve her English. Since most of her conversation may well be about how England is an economic desert and why can't you get fresh gnocchi at the grocers, or coy talks about 'my country', you may not be able to bear having her around. The point at which she turns up her nose at steak and kidney pie muttering about the exquisite taste of raw herrings rolled in vinegar is the time that she must go. She must also go the minute she gets pregnant, thrown in jail or all the other things that befall au pairs, because you will then feel you have *two* people to look after, rather than just one. The basic fault of au pairs is that your interests and theirs are different. They come to England to learn English and to have a good time; and you hire them to work and look after your child conscientiously. Because they are abroad au pairs tend to have little loyalty either to their jobs or to you. Being abroad exonerates them from all responsibility, it seems, and therefore you have to keep a very careful watch on them at all times.

They are also on a very uneasy footing in the household. They are, to a certain extent, one of the family because there they are, all vulnerable and foreign. And yet they're not likely to become real friends because they're too young, and are unlikely to want a personal relationship with you anyway. You will feel vaguely responsible for them all the time. Are they all right? Are they having 'a good time in England'?

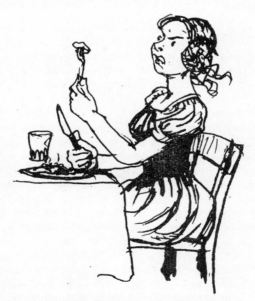

'She turns up her nose at steak and kidney pie'

However, many people have very successful au pairs, the most popular being the Dutch, Swedes, Germans and East Europeans. It helps to be totally impersonal and yet friendly, to give them a list of what they have to do and when they have to do it, and to make it absolutely clear when their time off is, and exactly what they can and cannot do in your house.

The biggest problem is that even when you get a winner, she will have to go just as she has consolidated a good relationship with your baby.

Nanny

It is hardly likely that you would employ a nanny to look after your baby while you go to work all day since you would probably have no money for yourself left over at all. She sometimes has the disadvantage of wanting to boss the parents around just as much as the children. But some mums have worked out excellent schemes where they share a nanny for, say, three afternoons a week when they all go off to work. This way you can be fairly sure of getting a good, reliable service with a woman who likes children and has enough experience to cope with any upsets.

Work while he sleeps

Sleep is the poor mother's au pair. Never use it. The minute you get down to doing anything constructive the baby will wake, howling.

Take the baby with you

And lose your job at once. Even if he is at the carrycot stage, this is rarely satisfactory.

Other mothers

The idea of baby-swaps is becoming more and more popular and your baby won't mind being left in a home similar to yours at all. The other mum could have yours on Mondays and you could have hers on Fridays. If you are swapping with someone you know and trust, it's worth putting up with any amount of initial screaming; the baby will soon settle down and become part of her family, as hers will become part of yours.

Remember that you are looking for someone for your baby and not for you. Usually the people you will get on with best may not be the ones your baby necessarily prefers. *He* may well adore some middle-aged granny with a permanently silly grin on her face. He may turn up his nose at long-skirted trendies with a good knowledge of pre-Raphaelite art and coo with delight at some lady of fifty who drones on and on about the price of butter, how great Enoch Powell is, whether baby's little handies are cold and someone who can remain, despite the five of her own she's reared, in perpetual astonishment at the number of teeth he has and what a wonderful baby he is. 'What a clever boy, aren't you a big boy, oh, you're a happy boy, what a clever boy, what a big boy.'

Whoever you leave him with must have your work phone number, the number of your GP and your partner's number.

When you've found someone to look after the baby, you then have to face the emotional gymnastics of leaving him, because while it may or may not be true that babies need their mums around when they are tiny, *lots* of mothers seem to need to be around their babies and feel painfully unhappy to be parted from them. The first time you go back to work or out to your evening class you will either find that when you arrive you feel you have never had a baby and that you can't remember what it is at home that you have to get back to, or you may feel you are still with the baby, hearing crying in your ears. As my arms hung all loose and lank by my side without the baby, I felt as if I'd left my handbag somewhere, a feeling of emptiness and loss that didn't help my work. It is a feeling something like arriving at work without your knickers. At least, I imagine it is. You're constantly aware of the draught, peculiarly uncomfortable and naked, even though you know that no one else can see and that it doesn't matter. People in the street don't even know you haven't got them on (or, rather, that you've left your baby behind) but you feel them staring at you all the same.

The only way to ameliorate the upsetting moment of parting is by visiting the person you are leaving the baby with several times with the baby before leaving him for the first time so that he gets to know the surroundings. And when you do finally go, *don't* dither; hanging about making things worse for everyone. Even if he's screaming, just give him a firm, confident kiss – and go, right away. *Then* you can burst into tears.

And make things easier on the baby by doing a good public relations job on the person you're leaving him with, too. Never under-pay, always over-pay. Remember presents for her birthday, or her children, because the more *she* feels part of your family, the more the baby will feel part of hers. And never try to interfere with her handling of your child. If you don't like her style, find someone else. You can't force someone to change their habits. She may be keen on dummies or extra cardigans or be over-fussy about cleanliness; or she may be a casual kind of person and you may be horrified to find your baby smiling when you return – but in unchanged nappies and with ice-cream all over his face. He will soon learn that what is okay at her place is not okay at yours, or vice-versa, and there is no reason to fear that he will expect you both to behave the same.

The mother who goes back to work will find herself the target of a mixture of disapproval and envy from those mothers who believe that staying at home is all-important. But if you believe that a happy mother helps to produce a (reasonably) happy baby, then you may have to go back to work some of the time, just to keep you both sane.

12

Baby Books

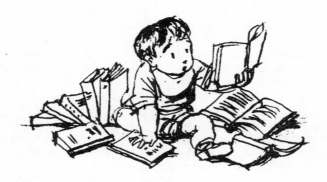

Like giving a child a Bible for its christening present or getting the complete Do-It-Youself Manual when moving into a new house, the first thing every mother does when she has a baby is to buy baby books. It's always thought that the latest baby book is the best book and these days baby books are thought to be more honest and liberal than they have ever been. The theories of Sir Frederick Truby King in 1940, for instance, are a marked contrast to Dr Hugh Jolly in 1975:

> 'Thumb-sucking: the best plan is to make a splint of corrugated cardboard. This allows free movement of the arm from the shoulder joint but prevents the hand from getting to the mouth. These splints should be taken off twice daily and the arms exercised and rubbed' (Sir Truby King: *Feeding and Care of Baby*, 1910).

> 'I dislike dummies because I would far prefer a baby who requires extra sucking to do it the natural way – by sucking his thumb' (Dr Hugh Jolly: *Book of Child Care*, 1975).

Mabel Liddiard's instruction in 1928 that 'The baby must *never* be taken into the nurse's or mother's bed' (*The Mothercraft Manual*) is confounded again by Dr Jolly: 'No harm results from bringing him [the baby] into the parental bed and parents will not be creating a rod for their backs as commonly feared.'

And compare: 'The waking of a baby to take food at any time between midnight and sunrise is unnatural' (Sir Frederick Truby King, *The Expectant Mother*, first edition 1916), with: 'A baby cannot be expected to last eight or so hours without being fed' (Dr Hugh Jolly in *Book of Child Care*). And what about: 'A newly born baby normally sleeps nine-tenths of its time. At six months it should sleep two-thirds of the time' (Sir Frederick Truby King in *Feeding and Care of Baby*), compared with: 'Few babies sleep through the night before six weeks' (Dr Miriam Stoppard, *Book of Babycare*, 1977).

Dr John Fairbairn, in *A Textbook for Midwives*, 1914, must have scared the daylights out of the new mother when he wrote:

> The careless, shiftless and ignorant mother whose child is brought up without method and given the breast whenever he cries for it is injuring both the health and character of her child. Not only is he likely to have disturbed digestion and irregularities in the action of the bowels, but he is acquiring the slipshod ways of his parents and without discipline and self-control he grows up self-willed and unable to adapt himself to our customs and is neither physically nor morally a credit to our race.

But I'm sure that some of the more liberal baby books of the sixties and seventies must have also taxed mothers to the hilt in their own, liberal way, urging them to be slave to their babies' every whim – with the added implications that if the mothers didn't care for them in the right way they would grow up to be, at best, simply suicidal, and, at worst, raving psychopaths.

Obviously we'd be inclined, these days, to agree more with an expert of today than one of 1910, particularly one called Truby. But the fact that the experts can disagree so drastically must make one wonder if, in the year 2000, another expert might come along to make the baby experts of today seem pretty foolish.

Baby books, however excellent, are only a poor substitute for a long talk with another sympathetic mother or doctor. But these days, with nuclear families, urbanised societies, lack of community spirit and all that, it's often difficult to find anyone to talk to at all. Baby books are much, much better than nothing. The mother alone in her flat with a small baby vomiting across the room and producing green stools in his nappies probably doesn't remember looking after a baby sister as her own mother might have done. Today's mothers have four walls and a telly and silence, and although the other mothers in the park with whom you will doubtless share all your fears and anxieties will be a considerable help, you'll find your best friends are new mothers; but for guidance and advice you need an older woman who has seen it all before (and yet not, of course, so much older that her theories are out of date).

Since the older generation that used to cope in times of crisis usually lives far away or has been brought up on the cries of routine feeding and believes that the 'continuous sucker' (of a dummy) 'is fortunate if he does not become a chain-smoker, a drunkard or a drug-addict' (Mrs Frankenburg, *Commonsense about Children*, 1970), we rely, naturally, on baby books.

The trouble with baby books is that while they reassure you about the worry you looked up in them, they worry you about something else in passing. Like a hypochondriac looking up 'peptic ulcer' in the medical dictionary when he's got a stomach-ache and finding that as well he's got phlebitis, pleurisy and polio, a mother will look up nappy rash and, just as she's closing the book with a sigh of relief, will spot a teeth chart and notice, to her horror, that most babies of her baby's age have four teeth and hers has not got one; and, to boot, it appears that he's a likely candidate for a cot death.

Baby books are, therefore, to be looked on sceptically. Even the jolliest, most reassuring ones (and even this one, come to that) can prompt usually normal women to crack with guilt or rage at a chance remark that, babyless, would leave them unaffected.

Then there are the baby book arguments. Baby books don't agree, even contemporary ones. Once your partner has got hold of one and you have got hold of another, you can spend evenings arguing and shouting like undergraduates at a union debate.

'Dr Spock says: "Put the baby to bed at a reasonable hour, say goodnight affectionately but firmly, walk out of the room and don't go back. Most babies who have developed this pattern cry furiously for twenty to thirty minutes the first night and then, when they see that nothing happens, they suddenly fall asleep!" So there!' announces your partner.

'Dr Spock has reneged on everything he's ever written!' you shriek back above the howls of the baby upstairs. 'You're mean and cruel! I must go to him! And Miriam Stoppard says: "In my opinion a baby should *never* be left to cry . . . if he is, he very soon realises that his pleas for attention go unheeded, that there is no loving, human response when he asks for it. What can happen then is that he stops asking and this may seriously damage his ability ever to form relationships with others!" I must go up and see what is wrong! Poor little boy!'

'Well, if you like, but I don't happen to agree with Dr Stoppard! And nor, as it happens, does Dr Spock. You're getting the child into bad habits and he must be trained out of them. Look, it says so here!' replies your partner, fumbling for the relevant page under Spoiling.

Collapse of mother into tears (and there are no mothers' books that will tell anyone what to do about this outburst) and no speaks for the rest of the night.

Both you and your partner will have *some* knowledge of handling babies, of course, simply from your own experiences – from your own parents' treatment of you when you were babies. And, hopefully, it will have been a good experience. The great danger is, if you have had a bad experience, to start treating the baby just as you were treated yourself. At best you will both be so confident that you will only need to use a baby-book for reference, when the baby falls ill. But most likely you *won't* be that confident. And when you read a baby book you'll find, even today, an idealistic view of motherhood.

If you're like me you'll want to skip books that give the kind of advice that makes you feel guilty. Avoid books that rave about birth and babies until you are confident that you are a raver too. There's nothing more depressing than reading about how a wonderful, loving, fulfilled and caring mother should behave when you don't feel a bit wonderful, loving, fulfilled or caring yourself. I've listed some good baby books at the end of the book.

Baby books these days still have romantic ideas about babies. They don't harp on about babies being 'sweet' or 'tender' as they used to. But they take babies very seriously and talk a lot about bonding and relationships and dependence. There's more to a baby than a rattle-waving gurgler who sleeps like a lamb and spends all day chuckling to himself in a cot. But there's also more to a baby than an earnest, serious relationship. Babies are erratic, they appear to be cruel, thoughtless, amoral, desperate, vulnerable, charming, cuddly, angelic, good and bad. To come to terms with a baby, if you're a new mother, is almost as difficult as trying to communicate with the weather.

But trying to grow anything requires delicate handling. And if even the best farmers always end up gloomily hanging over a gate complaining about the state of the sky, why should mothers be any different? Babies can't be grown from a book. There's no 'correct' baby any more than there's a perfect tree. You, the mother, cannot force a baby to be happy or sad; you can only try to help him to be himself . . . whatever that might be.

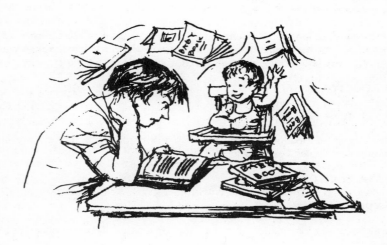

Further Help

NATIONAL CHILDBIRTH TRUST
Alexandra House, Oldham Terrace, Acton, London W3 6NH.
Telephone 01 992 8637

Advice, support, counselling in all aspects of childbirth, private classes, antenatal classes, breastfeeding and postnatal support. Leaflets available. Groups all over the country.

LA LECHE LEAGUE OF GREAT BRITAIN
BM 3424, London WC1N 6XX.
Telephone 01 404 5011; 24 hour 242 1278

Counsels on all aspects of breastfeeding.

ASSOCIATION OF BREASTFEEDING MOTHERS
131 Mayow Road, London SE26 4HZ.
Telephone 01 778 4769 for recorded message listing counsellors

Meetings with breastfeeding counsellors to discuss all aspects of breastfeeding and parenting. Newsletter and brochure in many languages.

ASSOCIATION FOR IMPROVEMENTS IN THE MATERNITY SERVICES (AIMS)
163 Liverpool Road, London N1 0RF.
Telephone 01 278 5628

Offers information, support and advice about all aspects of maternity care including rights for pregnant mothers ie choice in whether to have an episiotomy or not, choice about being given drugs, choice in delivery position.

MATERNITY ALLIANCE
15 Britannia Street, London WC1X 9JP.
Telephone 01 837 1265

Provides an information service for prospective parents, pregnant women and parents with babies. Leaflets available.

ACTIVE BIRTH CENTRE
55 Dartmouth Park Road, London NW5 1SL.
Telephone 01 267 3006

Leaflets, classes, information on active birth. Groups around the country.

SOCIETY TO SUPPORT HOME CONFINEMENT
Lydgate Lane, Walsingham, Co Durham DL13 3HA.
Telephone (after 6pm) 0388 5208044

Helps those who want a home birth but encounter obstructiveness or have problems making the necessary arrangements.

ASSOCIATION FOR THE ADVANCEMENT OF MATERNITY CARE
Sycamores, Chilbolton, Stockbridge, Hants.

Aims to make all kinds of pain relief available to women having babies.

THE MISCARRIAGE ASSOCIATION
PO Box 24, Ossett, West Yorks.
Telephone 0924 85515

Gives information and help after a miscarriage.

ASSOCIATION FOR POST-NATAL ILLNESS
7 Gowan Avenue, London SW6 6RH.
Telephone 01 731 4867

Countrywide network of volunteers who have recovered from post-natal depression.

CAESAREAN SUPPORT GROUP
7 Green Street, Willingham, Cambridge CB4 5JA.
Telephone 0954 60630

Monthly meetings, counselling and information. Leaflets available.

EARLYBIRTH ASSOCIATION
16 Warnham Rise, Hollingbury, Brighton, East Sussex BN1 8DF.
Telephone 0273 559634

Support group for mothers of premature babies.

CRYSIS
BM Crysis, London WL1N 3XX

National voluntary support group for mothers of crying babies. For practical advice and sympathetic understanding.
Send a S.A.E. or ring 01 404 5011 for your local number.

TWINS CLUBS ASSOCIATION (Twins and Multiple Births Association)
292 Valley Road, Lillington, Leamington Spa, Warwickshire CV32 7UE

Gives encouragement and support to parents of twins and multiple births.

MAMA (Meet-a-Mum Association)
Kate Goodyer, 3 Woodside Avenue, South Norwood, London SE25 5DW.
Telephone 01 654 3137

Self-help organisation for mothers of small children nationwide. Social gatherings, advice and support and also helps mums to find friends.

MOTHER AND BABY magazine runs a contacts page called 'In Touch'. Buy it and get in touch if you want to!

In all cases please enclose a S.A.E. if writing.

Australian Addresses

LA LECHE LEAGUE AUSTRALIA
c/o Pinky Mackay, 8 Gateshead Drive, Wantirna, Vic 3152, Australia

Counsels on all aspects of breastfeeding.

NURSING MOTHERS ASSOCIATION OF AUSTRALIA
PO Box 231, Nunawading, Vic 3131, Australia
Telephone 03 877 5011

The largest support group for breastfeeding mothers in Australia. Groups and counselling network, check your telephone book or contact their headquarters for your nearest branch.

PARENTS CENTRES AUSTRALIA
32 Station Street, Harris Park, NSW 2150, Australia
Telephone 02 633 5899

Parents' support group providing pre-natal classes and breastfeeding counselling.

COMMUNITY HEALTH CENTRES
Check in your local telephone book under Department of Health or Health Commission in the State Government section. These offer a wide variety of services, from home nursing and visits by midwives, to counselling, nutritional advice, psychologists and social workers.

BABY HEALTH CENTRES
INFANT WELFARE CENTRES
Operated by the Health Commission, check in your local telephone book.

AUSTRALIAN CHILDBIRTH EDUCATION AND PARENTING ASSOCIATION
PO Box 443, Ringwood, Vic 3134, Australia

For a complete list of childbirth education groups in Australia.

DIAL-A-MUM
Palmerston Road, Hornsby, NSW 2077, Australia
Telephone 02 477 6777

Telephone helpline for mothers who need a listening ear, advice or some social contact.

KARITANE MOTHERCRAFT SOCIETY
171 Avoca Street, Randwick, NSW 2031, Australia
Telephone 02 399 7086

Help for mothers with problem babies, either through their clinic, in-patient hospital or from mobile health clinics.

TRESILLIAN
Cnr Shaw Street and Addison Road, Petersham, NSW 2049, Australia
Telephone 02 569 5773

Help for mothers with difficult or problem babies. Phone counselling or residential and day care with expert assistance.

LONE PARENT FAMILY SUPPORT SERVICE
Cromer Community Centre, Cromer, NSW 2099, Australia
Telephone 02 982 1422

Support service for single parent families.

New Zealand Addresses

For addresses outside the Wellington area, contact your local Plunket Society or Social Services department.

PLUNKET SOCIETY
3 Moncrieff St, Mt Victoria, Wellington
Telephone 04 844 973

A nation-wide network of centres providing advice and assistance in all aspects of pregnancy, childbirth etc.

LA LECHE LEAGUE
Box 13 383, Wellington 4
Telephone 04 785 213

Support and advice for those wishing to breastfeed.

COT DEATH SUPPORT GROUP
Telephone 04 727 072

GEMINI CLUB
Telephone 04 887 847/837 518

A group that helps people with twins or multiple births.

MOTHERS HELPERS ASSOCIATION
Telephone 04 847 103/757 452

Home help for people under stress.

NEW ZEALAND PARENTS CENTRES
(Head office) Box 17-351, Karori, Wellington
Telephone 04 766 950

Offers a wide range of ante and post natal classes at a local level. Also some early childhood education, and coffee meetings for parents with children at home.

Booklist

Bourne, Gordon, *Pregnancy* (Pan 1984)
Jolly, Hugh, *Book of Child Care* (Unwin Hyman 1975)
Junor, Penny, *What Everywoman needs to Know* (Century 1988)
Kitzinger, Sheila, *Birth after Thirty* (Sheldon Press 1982)
Kitzinger, Sheila, *Birth at Home* (Oxford University Press 1980)
Leach, Penelope, *Babyhood* (Penguin 1983)